Designed by mshdesignspk@gmail.com

Edited by MountainCom LLC (mtcom@comcast.net)

Published by Audrey Burgio

www.exercisestrength.com

KETTLEBELL SPORT & FITNESS BASICS

PRINCIPLES, METHODOLOGY, TECHNIQUE TIPS, WORKOUTS & MORE

AUDREY BURGIO

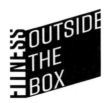

TABLE OF CONTENTS

INTRODUCTION

How My Journey Started

My fitness journey began around 2011. I saw an infomercial on TV advertising 10 minute workout videos that could be done at home. Just weeks prior, I was telling myself how I needed to be more active. I noticed I was putting on a little fat. I was the heaviest I had ever been and it worried me a little. Obesity, poor diet, and a lot of bad habits run rampant in my family. Seeing those videos felt like a sign that shouldn't be ignored. I ordered them without hesitation.

The videos arrived a few days later and I started doing one of the workouts every morning. Then, after a week or two, I started doing two of the videos each day. Moving my body felt good. I noticed an increase in my energy and mood. A few more weeks passed and I decided that I wanted to do more than just the videos.

I started taking a few dance classes. I have always found dancing appealing because it takes a combination of physical capacity and mental focus. I did that until I discovered "adult gymnastics" was a thing. Adult gymnastics consisted of learning new skills and they offered a workout after every class. I found that I loved the workout, which led me to seek a fitness specific class for the days I wasn't doing gymnastics. That is when I had found a style of group fitness called CrossFit.

In 2012, my coach at the time pushed me to start powerlifting and coaching classes myself. Two things happened at this point: first, I began learning how to coach. For me coaching came naturally. I was able to learn quickly how to assess proper movement and queue people in a variety of ways to elicit a specific result. I was coached to be a coach, while simultaneously starting my formal education relating to training people. Second, I started training and competing in powerlifting. I didn't train very long before doing my first competition. Jumping into a competition may sound crazy, but it set the tone for the rest of my fitness training. It made me realize that no one ever feels ready.

There is literally no amount of preparation you can do to ever feel "ready". Yes, you do want to train and plan for a competition in your training cycles, but you will likely never feel ready because there will always be a desire to do more, to be better. In my mind, what makes a competition successful is that you give 100%.

That's why it's a never-ending journey that keeps your attention. You show up, no matter where you are in your training and do the best you can. This was an invaluable lesson to learn early in my journey.

IF YOU DO THE BEST YOU CAN, THERE IS NO SPACE FOR DISAPPOINTMENT.

How I found Kettlebell Sport

After coaching Crossfit for a while I wanted to continue to learn skills and be a better coach in other disciplines. I found a class on teaching kettlebells in early 2013. At the time I had no idea kettlebell sport existed. I honestly had no idea what I would be learning. I assumed it would be your basic kettlebell movements like swings and presses.

I showed up to the class and learned more than I ever could have anticipated. People all across the world have competed in this sport for well over 50 years. Apart from being introduced to the sport-specific movements, I received coaching on numerous kettlebell exercises, including unfamiliar techniques like windmills and a variety grip positions that were previously unknown to me. The vast number of exercises and movements that can be done with a kettlebell was surprising.

During the class it was presented to us that there would be a casual competition the following weekend. The competition consisted of six different lifts each done for 10 minutes. What gave me the confidence to do the competition is that we would be able to choose our weight, set the kettlebells down, and switch hands as needed. That next weekend, I was lifting the lightest weights there were (8kg), but it didn't matter. I did all the lifts. It was challenging and also very rewarding. The competition was exciting to me because, similar to dance and gymnastics, it takes physical and mental tenacity. I was hooked.

2020 Gym Closures and Obstacles

When most of the gyms closed during 2020, it was an easy transition to take my kettlebells outside or workout inside my tiny studio apartment. That first kettlebell competition inspired me. By 2020, I had earned coaching certifications from CrossFit, IKLF, USAKL, Kettacademy and ISSA for kettlebell coaching, personal fitness training, bodybuilding and endurance. I had my kettlebells and I knew how to get a full body workout. I had no excuses. I created a program for myself to follow, much like the one in this book. I would be on the sidewalk, rain or shine. People would walk by and cheer me on, or share how motivating it was to see me out there almost everyday. I was able to encourage my neighbor to work out too. Realizing how many people needed help during this time encouraged me to put more effort into my Fitness Outside The Box program.

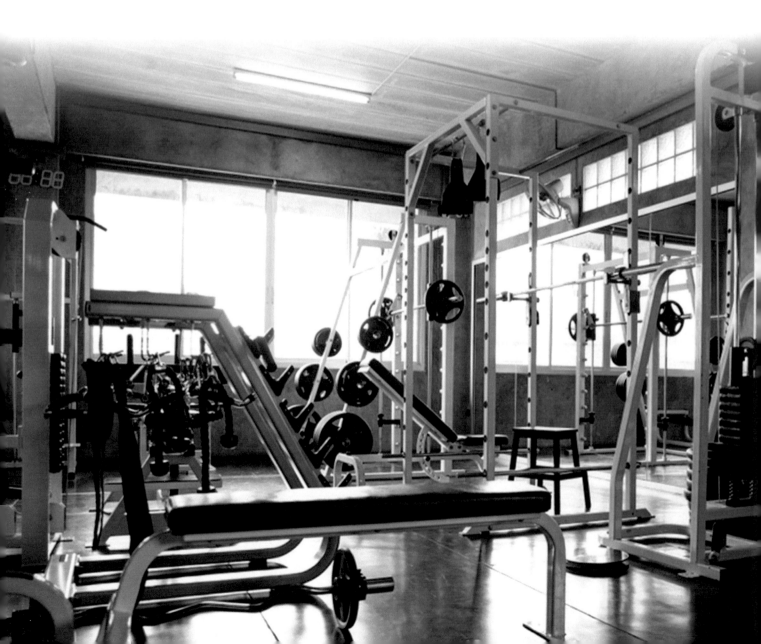

Fitness Outside The Box is a no-excuse approach to training. There's always a way to get an effective workout no matter where you are or what equipment you have available. Let's talk about excuses. You have the time because you make the time. Anything you want to progress at must become a priority. It could be working out, gaining muscle, living a healthier lifestyle, learning a new computer program or cooking. Whatever it is, it must be important to you. You are likely to make going to work a priority, your goals need to be a priority as well. There should be no difference in your mind between work and your goals. You schedule your goal in and you follow through no matter what. There has to be some level of perseverance with everything you do. You have to hold yourself accountable. You are only cheating and lying to yourself when you don't follow through on the commitments you make to yourself. No one else is going to care if you don't go to the gym or eat poorly.

It is paramount that you pick small and achievable goals. This allows you to stay focused, not get discouraged, and build trust with yourself. If you spent the last decade or more eating terribly, partying, not exercising, don't all of a sudden try eating salads everyday, not going out for drinks and telling yourself you are going to go to the gym everyday. That will be quite the challenge and likely not be sustainable. Yes, it can work to make drastic changes and stick to them. But it doesn't work for the majority of people. Let's say your goal is to be healthier and nothing you currently do is healthy. You need to pick a few things to focus on. You do those few things for a couple weeks to a month and then you add in more. I recommend picking three things.

If you are in the situation I described above where you are eating bad, drinking too much alcohol and not doing anything physical for your body here are three examples of things you can start with:

- You could choose to cut your alcohol consumption by half. So, instead of eight drinks a week you commit to only having four.
- Let's say you have a sweet tooth and eat a lot of sugar. You could commit to only consuming natural sugars like honey and fruit (in moderation).
- You could ride your bike for 20 minutes after work, take a group fitness class, or get on the treadmill while you watch a TV show.

Say you do those few changes for 14 days. By the end of the first week, you'll feel pretty good if you stick to your plan. For the most part, it doesn't matter what the "plan" is. What matters is that you stick to it.

There will come a time in your journey when you'll need to change course or have a more focused approach, but small steps are where you should start. Another quick example: Let's say you want to do a pull-up. You currently can't do one. You have no idea how to begin, so you get discouraged. So what do you do?

Of course, the answer is not "nothing." There are hundreds of videos online that can show you how to scale pull-ups and build the strength you need to achieve doing one. You can start out practicing every day, or at least a few times a week. Depending on your fitness level, body weight, age and starting strength, this could take a few weeks or a few months. But it doesn't matter how long. You work that goal until you get it.

There was a time years ago when one of my goals was to do a muscle-up on the rings. A muscle-up is where you do a pull-up, turn your hands over, and then do a dip. The best I could do was about 3-5 pull-ups and a couple dips. I asked a coach at the gym to give me a few pointers on the muscle-up. He showed me where to place my hands, when to turn them over, and how I should position my body. At first it still seemed impossible. I could do a pull-up, but when I would go to do the second part of the movement, my body simply did not know what to do. But I spent the next six months practicing. Every day when I got to the gym, I practiced the skill for 5-10 minutes. I would do jumping muscle-ups, working on pulling the rings to my chest. I worked on my ring dips. I worked on every phase of the exercise, and finally the day came when I completed the movement.

There is something really special about achieving a goal at the end of a long road of commitment and dedication. The size of the goal doesn't matter; it can be drinking a gallon of water every day, not eating sugar for one day, not getting on social media for a few hours, or flossing your teeth. It doesn't matter.

It's all about your mindset. So, what's the correct mindset to have at the gym or when you're working out? When you start a workout, you need to finish it. It's okay if some days you're feeling tired and move a little slower or work with lighter weights. But you're still finishing the workout. Obviously, there are exceptions to this rule, but they're rare: something starts aching, or you have limited time so you decide to get as far as you can in the time you have. Life happens. But that should not stop you from staying dedicated to what you're doing.

Let's say you decide to do a 12-minute cardio circuit. You're 8 minutes in and feeling a little tired or bored. Don't stop at 9 or 10 minutes in. Finish it no matter what. When you do what you said you would do, you feel accomplished and proud, and you build integrity. As I mentioned before, you need to give

100% effort to everything you do — from making your bed to finishing your workout. These are the habits that separate you from the majority of people. They are not difficult habits to form, but as you stick with them they'll become even easier until you find yourself doing them automatically.

Celebrate the small victories along the way, acknowledging that each step, regardless of its size, contributes to the bigger picture. Embrace the journey with the understanding that consistency and perseverance, no matter how incremental, lay the foundation for meaningful progress. Whether it's a daily fitness routine, a nutritional commitment, or a personal wellness goal, the mindset of continuous effort and completion fosters a sense of accomplishment and fuels the motivation to tackle even more significant challenges.

WHAT MATTERS IS THAT YOU STICK TO WHAT YOU'VE TOLD YOURSELF YOU'RE GOING TO DO.

KETTLEBELL SPORT & FITNESS BASICS

Why Train with Kettlebells

Kettlebell training provides a challenging and effective workout that can help to improve physical and mental fitness. Kettlebell exercises are often dynamic and multi-joint movements that engage multiple muscle groups at once, making it an efficient and effective full-body workout. Many kettlebell exercises are high-intensity, which raise your heart rate and improve your cardiovascular fitness. Kettlebell training can increase strength and power, especially in the lower body and core.

Many kettlebell exercises require a high level of stability and balance, which can help to improve overall balance and stability in everyday life. Kettlebell training can help to increase range of motion and flexibility in the hips, shoulders, and spine. Kettlebells are relatively small and easy to store, making them a versatile piece of equipment that can be used for a variety of exercises and training styles. Kettlebell training can be mentally challenging, especially during high-intensity exercises, which can help to build mental toughness and resilience.

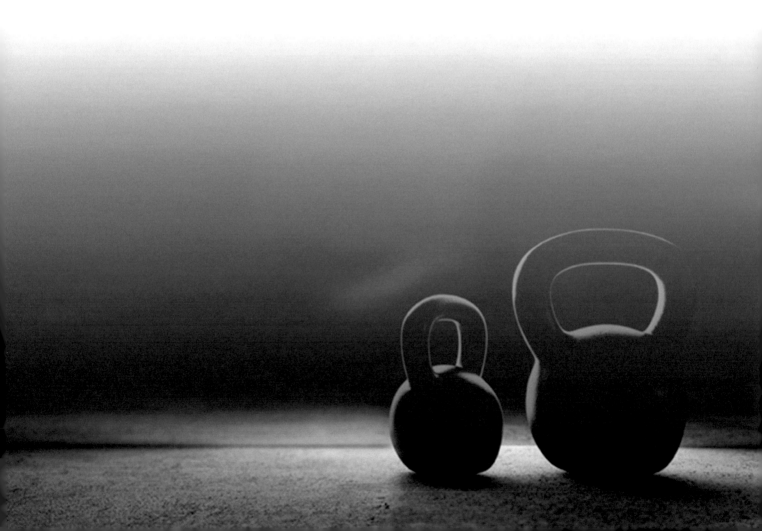

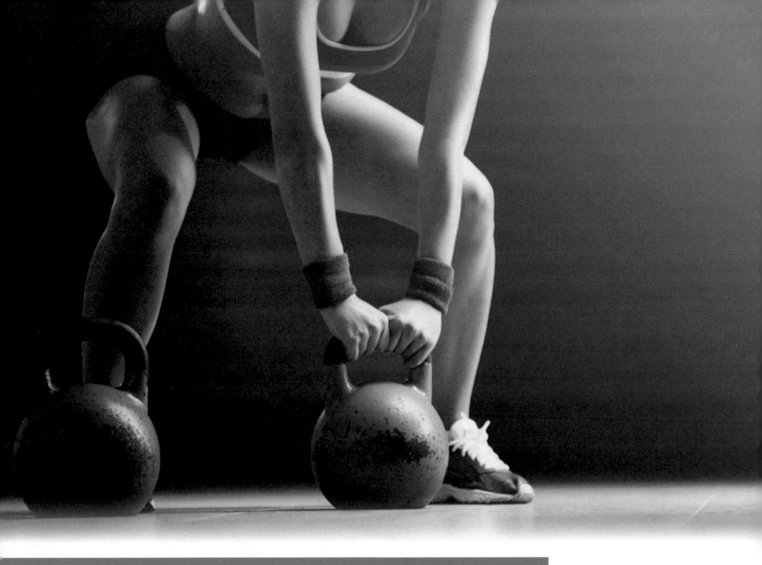

Why I Created This KB Training Program

The program in this book will allow you to get an effective training session, regardless of your fitness level or experience. All you need to complete the workouts are a few kettlebells and a band. If you don't have kettlebells or bands yet you can easily find what you need online.

For the bands, I recommend getting a variety of sizes. They are often sold in packs of three or five and are very affordable. If you search for "pull up band" that will bring up the same style shown in this program. For the kettlebells, I recommend a competition-style kettlebell. It is best to have a variety of weights and, if your budget allows, having two kettlebells of the same weight. The more variety you have the better.

You can do the workouts in the comfort of your home or take the program to the gym with you. By following the program, you will learn how easy it is to get an effective workout with minimal equipment regardless of where you train. Don't let excuses stop you.

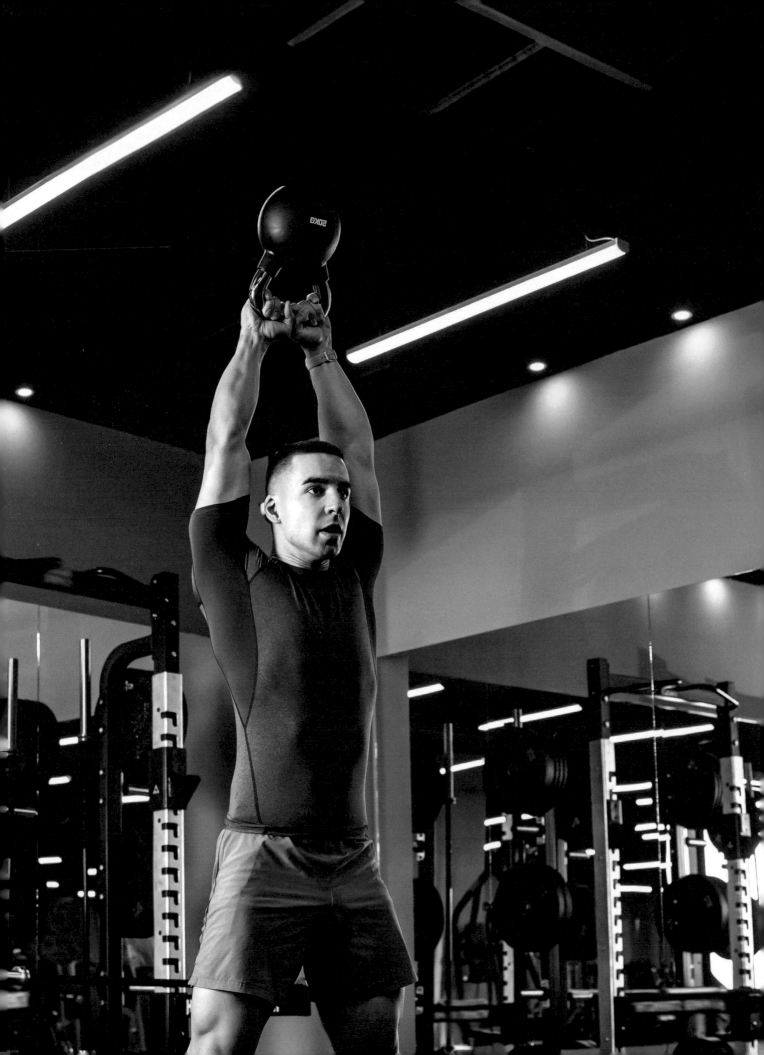

PLEASE NOTE

The information presented in this guide is basic. I've tried to take complex concepts that have many variables and make them simple. There is no one perfect training system. My intention is to give you enough information to be successful in starting your new fitness journey or add to your existing one.

It is recommended that you consult with your physician before beginning any exercise program. You should be in good physical condition and be able to participate in exercise. When participating in any exercise or exercise program, there is the possibility of physical injury. If you engage in exercise or an exercise program, it is at your own risk. By participating in these activities, you assume all risk of injury to yourself, and agree to release Audrey Burgio, Exercisestrength.com, Fitness Outside the Box, and all other affiliates from any and all claims or causes of action, known or unknown, arising out of any negligence. The views and opinions expressed here within are exactly that, views and opinions.

FITNESS BASICS

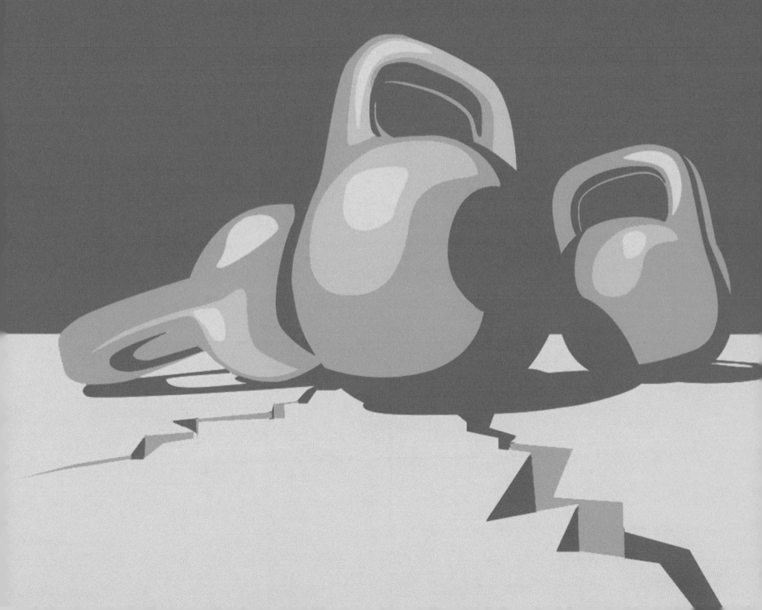

THE KETTLEBELL

There are two main types of kettlebells: standard and competition. Standard kettlebells vary in their shapes, sizes, and materials, with options ranging from cast iron to vinyl or plastic. As the weight of the standard kettlebell increases, so does its overall size.

In contrast, competition-style kettlebells adhere to a uniform size and shape and are hollow on the inside. The size of the core determines the weight of the kettlebell, and they are often distinguished by standard colors.

Non-competition kettlebells have a slightly rounder and larger window, providing more space for a two-handed grip. On the other hand, competition kettlebells feature a more rectangular handle design that allows the hand to sit comfortably inside. These competition kettlebells typically have narrower and uniform handle diameters, which enhance grip endurance. Most competition style kettlebells have similar handle shapes and sizes but the various brands do differ slightly and you'll probably discover your preference after trying a few out.

Additionally, the steel handle on a competition kettlebell allows for better chalk absorption, ensuring a firmer grip, and its smoother surface reduces friction during high-repetition movements. Competition kettlebells exhibit a more balanced weight distribution between the handle and the base which enhances stability in a variety of positions.

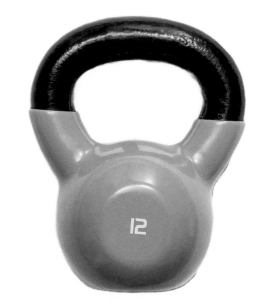

While the exercises in this program and book can be performed with either style of kettlebell, it is advisable to use the competition style due to its larger base providing increased stability during exercises that involve the kettlebell resting on the floor.

Personal preference and comfort play a crucial role in choosing the right kettlebell for your workouts. Experimenting with both styles can help you determine which one aligns better with your fitness goals and feels more comfortable during various exercises.

STANDARD KETTLEBELL

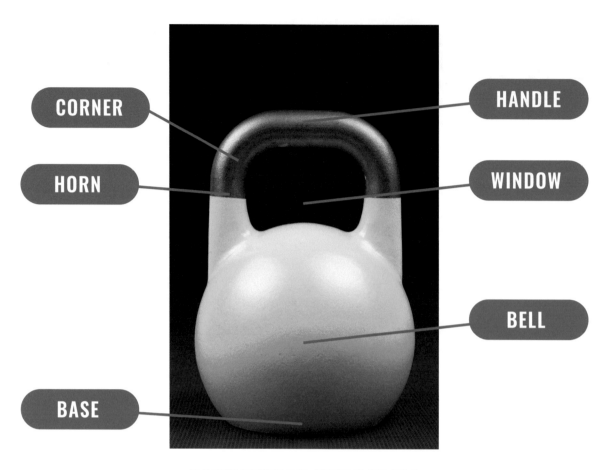

CORNER

HANDLE

HORN

WINDOW

BELL

BASE

COMPETITION KETTLEBELL

Color	Kg	Lb
Pink	8	18
Blue	12	26
Yellow	16	35
Purple	20	44
Green	24	53
Orange	28	62
Red	32	70
Gray	36	79
White	40	88
Silver	44	97
Gold	48	106

TRAINING TIPS

Prioritize your lifting technique

Your main focus should always be on technique - not weight and reps. As your technique improves, you'll find yourself completing more reps and lifting heavier weights. Prioritizing technique will help reduce your risk of injury and increase your overall strength. Remember, quality movements lay the foundation for sustainable progress in your fitness journey.

Practice the full range of motion of each exercise

Perform each exercise through its full range of motion. If your range of motion is deficient in any areas due to a lack of mobility, work specifically on those during warm-up and cool-down. For example, if you're unable to squat below parallel due to tight hips, warm up with goblet squats as shown on page 75, incorporate dynamic hip stretches into your warm-up routine, and dedicate time during the cool-down for static stretches to gradually improve hip flexibility and address any mobility limitations.

Rest between sets

Resting between sets is important regardless of your fitness experience. Rest 2-4 minutes or as long it takes for your muscles to almost function at full capacity again (restore depleted energy). Adequate rest intervals prevent the accumulation of fatigue within a set which can enable you to maintain proper form and technique. For example, if your program has you doing 8 reps of squats for 5 sets, rest at least 2 minutes after your 8 squats. Lighter weight or lower-effort movements will take less time to restore your energy stores. Note: You'll know you're recovered when you feel ready to do the next set, your heart rate has lowered and your muscles have stopped burning from your last set. Keep in mind though, that some programmed sets will explicitly call for less rest depending on the phase of training.

Allow yourself time to recover

Ensure you're recovering from one workout day to the next. Over-training or overuse will result in injury, so listen to your body. Everyone recovers differently. You'll know you're ready for your next workout when you have good energy and your muscles aren't excessively sore from your previous session.

Video yourself

Record your sets and analyze your form regularly. Use slow motion occasionally for a more detailed look. Video review will provide immediate feedback, which is important for progression. Your average cell phone will do the trick. This visual feedback not only helps in identifying areas for improvement but also serves as a valuable tool for tracking your progress over time. By regularly reviewing your recorded sets, you can make informed adjustments to your technique, ensuring continued growth and refinement in your training journey.

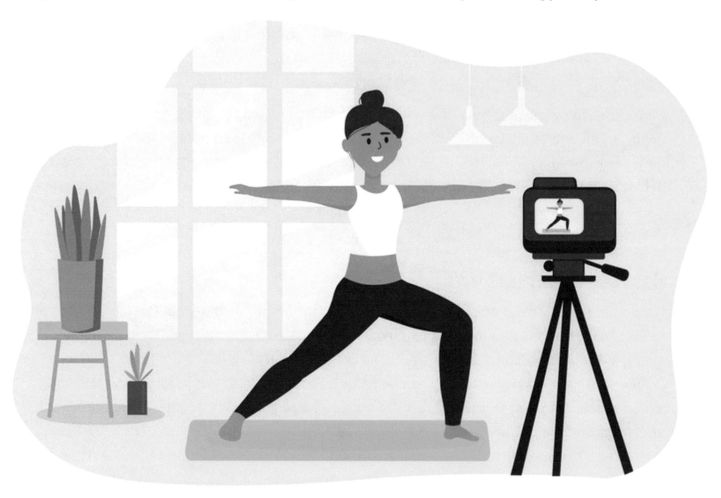

Track and record your workouts

Keep a record of your workouts. Write down the weight you used, the time it took, and even how if felt. Keeping track of your workouts will help guide you to pick the correct weights and intensity for future sessions. I recommend using a spreadsheet or writing in a notebook. There is a sample workout log at the end of this book you can photocopy. You can also find a free printable version online at www.exercisestrength.com/products.

PRINCIPLES AND METHODOLOGY

CONSIDER THESE 5 AREAS WHEN TRAINING TO MAXIMIZE RESULTS AND CREATE A BALANCED BODY

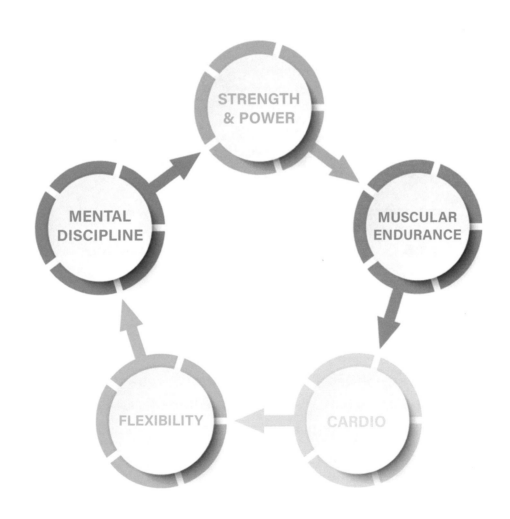

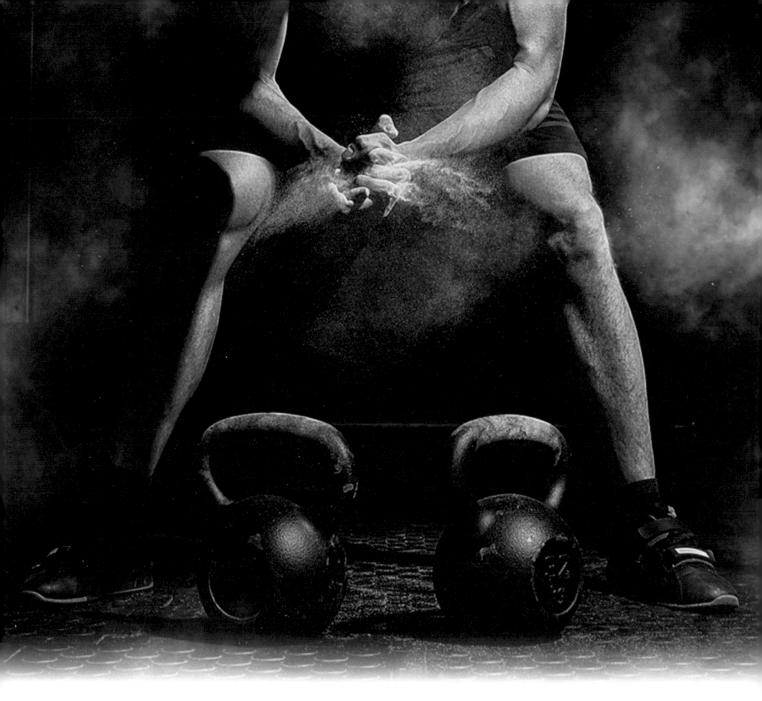

Strength & Power

Strength and power differ slightly but are closely related. Because one directly affects the other, I've grouped them together here. Strength can be defined as the application of muscular force to overcome resistance. Power is measured as force exerted over time. Strength plus speed equals power. It's important to build a solid base of strength by weightlifting. Once a foundation of strength is established, then power and acceleration can be trained more effectively. Integrating compound exercises such as squats, deadlifts, and bench presses into your weightlifting regimen contributes to a holistic enhancement of overall strength by engaging multiple muscle groups. As your strength advances, incorporate explosive movements that emphasize the synergy of strength and speed, aiming to specifically enhance power and acceleration.

Muscular Endurance

Your ability to contract muscles repeatedly over an extended period of time (complete more reps) will directly affect your muscles' aerobic capacity and increase your athletic performance—both of which are critical for kettlebell sport. Aerobic capacity measures your maximum oxygen consumption during physical activity. During high-intensity activities, your cardiac output increases as your body requires more oxygen to keep performing. As you do aerobic exercises more regularly, your aerobic capacity will increase. Circuit training is a great and an effective way to enhance overall muscular endurance and fitness. Incorporating diverse exercises within a circuit further ensures a comprehensive approach to fitness, making it an efficient and engaging way to elevate both muscular endurance and overall fitness levels.

Cardio

Aerobic exercise provides cardiovascular training. Aerobic training is any form of exercise that uses oxygen for the production of energy. The lungs bring oxygen into the body to provide energy and the heart pumps oxygen to the muscles. Your aerobic fitness level directly impacts the supply of much-needed oxygen to your muscles, as well as the carrying away of metabolic waste products like carbon dioxide and lactic acid. Aerobic training helps the body more efficiently take oxygen through the lungs and pump it to the muscles. Cardiovascular training offers benefits to athletes across all different levels.

Flexibility & Mobility

Sufficient flexibility is necessary to address daily activities and training requirements, with an additional margin to handle unforeseen situations such as slipping on ice or falling. Start by working the areas you're most deficient in. Achieving proper positioning in the lifts is critical to being efficient and injury free. You must develop strength, flexibility and stability concurrently in order to have strength in the new range of motion. Failure to strengthen the end range is an invitation for injury and a substantial reduction in force output ability. When faced with poor mobility or stability, it's essential to modify movements as needed.

Mental Discipline

Set goals and commit to training. Make sure your initial goals are realistic and achievable. If you're not consistent and committed, you won't see the results you want. Consistency leads to self-discipline, which leads to accountability. Consistency also fosters a positive feedback loop, reinforcing the habit of regular training and making it easier to stay on track. Celebrate small victories along the way to maintain motivation and momentum.

HABITS
TO CONSIDER
ADOPTING

Drink water first thing in the morning

Drinking water first thing in the morning is important for several reasons. When you sleep you can become dehydrated. Hydrating first thing in the morning will give you a great head start on staying hydrated all day. Proper hydration also helps with digestion (it detoxifies the liver and kidneys, and carries waste away). Try for at least 16oz as soon as you roll out of bed. Keep a full glass next to your bed so it is ready for you when you wake.

Eat a diet rich in color

Eating a variety of different-colored foods will ensure you're getting all the vitamins and minerals your body needs to function at its optimal level. Most of your daily vitamin and mineral requirements can be found in food through a balanced diet. You may want to consider asking your doctor or nutritionist if there are any micronutrients (vitamins and minerals) you should focus on, and whether supplements could be helpful for you. Various affordable micronutrient tests are available, providing an easy and cost-effective way to assess your nutrient levels.

Don't obsess over counting calories

When you stop eating processed foods and eat the right balance of protein, fat, and carbs, you can lose weight without having to count anything. Each meal should consist of protein, healthy fats, and carbohydrates. Tracking your meals using a macronutrient calculator or following a meal plan can be helpful in getting you on the right track or reaching more specific bodyweight goals. Remember, the key to successful weight management lies not only in the nutritional composition of your meals but also in cultivating a healthy relationship with food that aligns with your individual lifestyle and preferences.

Have a schedule

Create a schedule and stick to it. Add in the things you want to get done, and follow through. Having a consistent routine will create healthy habits. Start out with small items and then add a new task as soon as you feel the previous tasks have become automatic. Set yourself up for success by utilizing the resources readily available to you for assistance, whether it's your phone or a notebook.

Rest and recovery

Make time to rest and recover. Recovery is an integral part of any program as it allows your muscles to repair themselves from previous training sessions. There are also important neurological and nervous system repairs that occur when you rest. Incorporating rest and recovery into your routine is crucial for optimizing overall performance and preventing burnout. A well-balanced program includes both exertion and recovery, creating a sustainable foundation for long-term health and fitness.

THE KEYS TO BEING SUCCESSFUL WITH ANY FITNESS PROGRAM ARE DISCIPLINE, SELF-REFLECTION, AND CONSISTENCY

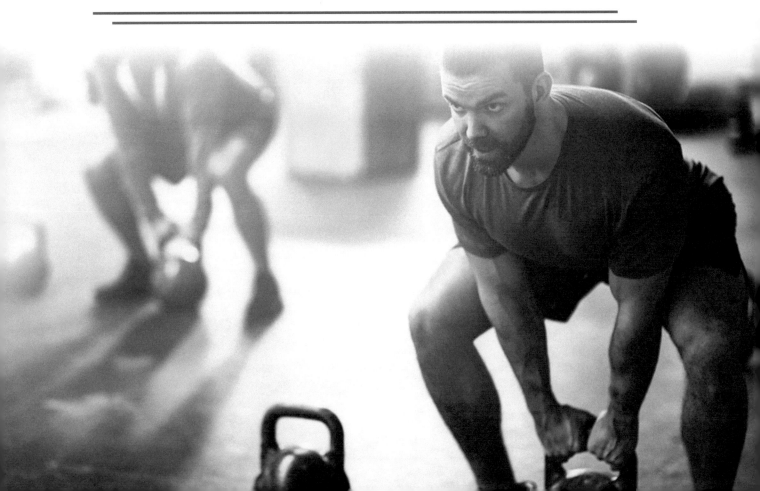

HOW MANY REPS?

Muscles respond differently to various types of exercise and load, making it essential to tailor your workout routine based on your fitness goals. The table below provides a fundamental repetition [rep] range to follow, depending on what your training focus is.

Benefits Produced	Reps
Speed	1 - 10
Strength	1 - 15
Hypertrophy	10 - 20
Strength Endurance	15 - 20+

The table below demonstrates how the quantity of reps or time duration will impact your specific training goal. The final repetition in whatever rep range you're working in should be performed at or near maximum effort.

Objective	Repetitions 1 → 15 → 30+				
Speed	Very High	High	Medium	Low	Very Low
Strength	High	Very High	High	Medium	Low
Hypertrophy	Low	Medium	Very High	High	Medium
Strength Endurance	Very Low	Low	Medium	Very High	Very High
	:01 → :45 → :90+				
	Time (seconds)				

Definition of Terms

Speed: The distance an object traveled compared to the time required to go that distance [1]

Strength: The ability to exert force

Power: The ability of a muscular unit, or combination of muscular units, to apply maximum force in minimum time [2]

Strength Endurance: The ability of muscles to repeatedly exert force against resistance [3]

Hypertrophy: The increase in muscle fiber size

Anaerobic: In the absence of oxygen

Aerobic: In the presence of oxygen

"Success is no accident. It is hard work, perseverance, learning, studying, sacrifice, and most of all, love of what you are doing or learning to do." - Pelé

[1] Wiki Targeted (Entertainment). (n.d.-b). Athlepedia, the Athletics Wiki. https://athletics.fandom.com/wiki/Speed

[2] Wiki Targeted (Entertainment). (n.d.). Athlepedia, the Athletics Wiki. https://athletics.fandom.com/wiki/Power

[3] Brown, E. (2019, July 17). What Is the Definition of Muscular Endurance? LIVESTRONG.COM. https://www.livestrong.com/article/392246-what-is-the-definition-of-muscular-endurance/

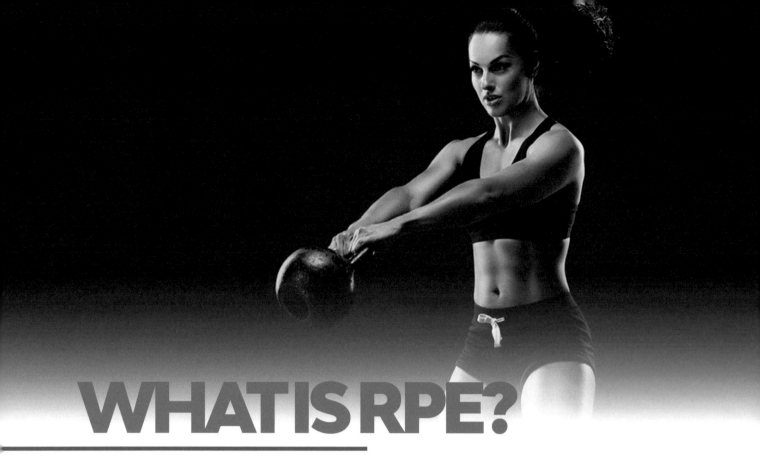

WHAT IS RPE?

RPE (rated perceived exertion) is a scale used to measure the perceived (subjective) intensity of your exercise. There are several RPE scales, each serving a specific purpose in assessing perceived exertion during various activities. Each of these scales serves as a tool to communicate and quantify your perceived exertion during physical activity, aiding in the assessment and monitoring of exercise intensity. It typically goes from 1-10, but can also be seen as 6-20, 0-20, or even 0-100. I recommend using the 1-10 scale. Recording the RPE of your workouts, at least your kettlebell sport training, will help you make sure you're not constantly over (or under) exerting yourself. We want a balance and a variety of training intensities. Some workouts will be designed for recovery and some for high intensity high heart rate.

RPE	Breathing/Exertion	MAX HR % (approximate)
1	Extremely Easy	50%
2 - 3	Very Easy	55% - 65%
4 - 6	Easy to Moderate Effort	65% - 75%
7 - 8	Moderately Difficult to Hard	75% - 85%
9	Very Hard	85% - 95%
10	Extremely Hard	95% - 100%

Record the RPE of your kettlebell, cardio, or HIIT* sessions in your workout notes. If you use a heart rate monitor, keep track of your heart rate too. I recommend writing down the max and average of each segment of your training. The more data you have, the better. Recording both your RPE and heart rate offers a few benefits:

1. You'll start to learn the correlation of RPE to heart rate, and will then be able to make adjustments to your sets on the fly.

2. You'll have data to track your progress and fitness level over time. You can look back at similar past training sessions and use that information to determine when to change your pace or weight.

3. You'll learn how to regulate your heart rate to maximize your volume output. Regulating your heart rate will help you avoid burning out too early.

For weightlifting, you'll generally focus on the 6 to 10 range on the scale. If your goal is strength, you would typically be in the 8-10 RPE range. A 10 RPE would be a max effort set. For hypertrophy, you would be in the 7-8 RPE range. Adjust the weights you are using based on your RPE ratings. If a set feels too easy, you can increase the weight. If it feels too challenging for the type of work you are doing, consider reducing the weight or taking longer rest intervals. It's important to tailor your approach to align with your fitness objectives and gradually progress within the recommended intensity zones to optimize your training outcomes.

Leverage the RPE scale as a powerful ally on your journey towards progress, as each recorded step is a testament to your dedication and a roadmap to your success!

*HIIT: High-Internsity Interval Training

Themes, U. (2017, May 22). Perceived Exertion Scaling Procedures. Musculoskeletal Key. https://musculoskeletalkey.com/perceived-exertion-scaling-procedures/

LEVELS OF
PROGRESSION

THE DREYFUS MODEL OF SKILL ACQUISITION

The Dreyfus model is used to assess and support progress in the development of a skill or competency. In the table below, I've adapted the Dreyfus model slightly for use in kettlebell sport and fitness. Just like in any sport or skill, it's important to learn and master the fundamentals before progressing to the next level. Understanding where you are can provide awareness, motivation, and a sense of direction. This foundational knowledge not only builds a solid base but also fosters a deeper appreciation for the intricacies of the activity. As you grasp the fundamentals, you gain confidence in your abilities, creating a sturdy platform from which to advance and tackle more advanced techniques with greater proficiency.

Level/Stage	Characteristics	Action
Novice	Needs supervision and/or instruction	Focus on consistency of one part of the lift over reps, pace, or weight
Advanced Beginner	Possesses a working understanding and can complete simpler tasks without supervision	Focus on consistency of the entire lift over reps, pace, or weight
Competent	Has a good working understanding; sees actions and understands them; able to complete work independently to a standard that is acceptable, though it may lack refinement	Start introducing more complex parts of the lift (i.e., methodical breathing, weight shifting, self-analysis)
Proficient	Possesses a deep understanding, views actions holistically, achieves a high standard routinely	Focus on maintaining form, pace, and efficiency as weight and heart rate increase
Expert	Possesses an authoritative or deep holistic understanding, able to deviate and perform tasks intuitively, able to go beyond existing interpretations, achieves excellence with ease	Focus on continual technique refinement, lift and train intuitively The 'expert' level does not signify that development stops, as expert practitioners need to evaluate their practice regularly

Adapted from: Dreyfus, Stuart E., Formal Models vs Human Situational Understanding: Inherent limitations on the Modeling of Business Expertise. USAF office of Scientific Research, Ref F49620-79-C-0063:. Extracts taken from devmts.org.uk/dreyfus.pdf and www-personal.umicH.edu/~mrotHer/kata_files/dreyfus.pdf

KETTLEBELL SPORT BASICS

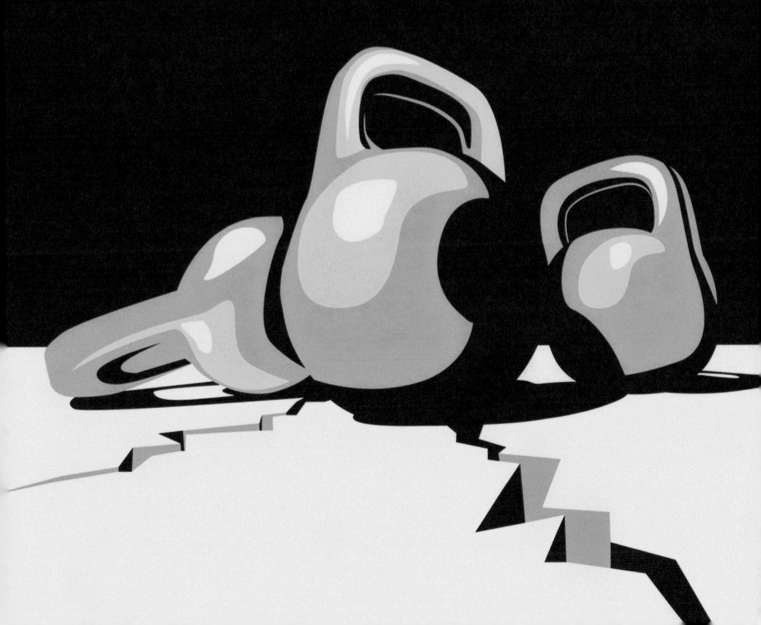

WHAT IS KETTLEBELL SPORT?

Kettlebell sport is an endurance weightlifting sport. Athletes are given points for each repetition completed during a timed set for both single and double kettlebell events. These timed sets can vary but are most often 10 minutes. Success in kettlebell sport demands a combination of strength, muscular endurance, efficiency, and a strong cardiovascular foundation. Reps or points are counted when the athlete achieves a "lockout" or "fixation." This occurs when the kettlebell has stopped moving overhead and the arms, hips, and legs are fully extended.

Athletes participate in categories based on their gender, age, and weight class. This ensures fair competition by grouping individuals with similar physical characteristics. Athletes within the same weight class lift kettlebells of the same weight during competitions.

Most lifting federations recognize the following lifts, or some combination thereof, for competition:

- Snatch
- Half Snatch
- Double Half Snatch
- Long Cycle
- Two-Arm Long Cycle
- Jerk
- Double Jerk

There are two primary sport types - Russian Girevoy and American BOLT. And, within the two styles there are many different lifting federations, events, and rankings. Athletes often strive to achieve specific rankings within their chosen federation, working towards personal goals and recognition within the kettlebell sport community. This diversity within the sport allows individuals to find their niche and compete in a manner that aligns with their strengths and preferences.

Russian

The inception of Girevoy sport [GS] competitions dates back to the 1940s. By the 1970s, it was integrated into the United All-State Sport Association of the USSR, having been introduced in educational institutions years prior. In 1981, the USSR government established an official commission endorsing kettlebell training for enhancing workforce fitness and productivity. This led to the formal recognition of Girevoy sport as a competitive activity with defined rules and regulations by 1985. In a standard Girevoy sport [GS} style competition, lifts are performed for a maximum of ten minutes.

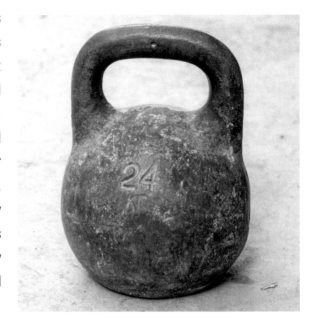

Lifters compete against others that are in the same weight class, lifting the same weight kettlebell. During the set, athletes complete as many reps as possible without placing the kettlebells on the ground. In single-arm events athletes are only allowed to switch hands one time. The lifter with the highest number of reps is the winner.

There are variations in the events offered during GS competitions but typically a competition consists of Long Cycle, Snatch Only, and Biathlon events. Biathlon is an event where lifters compete in both snatch and jerk.

The kettlebell weights used in most competitions are 16kg, 20kg, 24kg, 28kg, and 32kgs for men and 8kg, 12kg, 16kg, 20kg, and 24kg for women. Some national and international competitions are divided into only two categories, amateur and professional. Amateur men use the 24kg kettlebells while amateur woman use the 16kg. Professional men use the 32kg kettlebells, and professional women use the 24kg. There are also marathon events of 30 and 60 minutes that are often held at GS competitions.

Cotter, S. (2022) History of kettlebell and Kettlebell Sport, Human Kinetics. Available at: https://us.humankinetics. com/blogs/excerpt/history-of-kettlebell-and-kettlebell-sport (Accessed: 12 June 2022).

English, N. (2023) Kettlebell history goes back much further than Russia, BarBend. Available at: https://barbend. com/kettlebell-history/ (Accessed: 14 August 2023).

American

The kettlebell lifting sport known today as BOLT, got its start under the name American Rules Kettlebell Sport [ARKS} in 2009. BOLT fulfilled the need for a kettlebell sport that represented the American value of gender equality and the need to have a non-elitist, lifter-oriented sport. BOLT is like its counterpart, Russian Girevoy, with the exception that in the American version both men and women could compete in all the lifts – doubles and singles. International Kettlebell

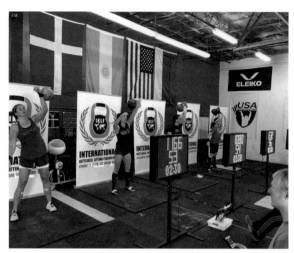

Lifting Federation [IKLF] was the first governing body to rule in favor of gender equality at a time when women weren't allowed to lift doubles by any of the other existing kettlebell sport governing organizations. Like ARKS, BOLT allows women to lift doubles. Now, many other federations allow woman to lift in all events. However, there are still some limitations on what weight kettlebells can be used. BOLT Kettlebell Lifting Sport diverted even farther from Russian Girevoy by eliminating the "one switch" rule and allowing for unlimited set downs and multiple hand switches.

BOLT allows lifters the flexibility to choose their own competition weights and lifts. BOLT Kettlebell Lifting Sport measures the lifter's overall work capacity by tallying the total amount of kilograms lifted during a set. In BOLT, lifters compete in the three single lifts, the three double lifts, or all six lifts in one day.

KETTLEBELL SPORT RANKING TABLES 201

WOMEN SNATCH

ght Cate-es (kg)	47	50	53	58	58+	63	63+	68	68+	KB Wei
SIC	–	–	110	120	–	130	–	140	150	24k
MS	–	–	90	100	–	110	–	120	130	20k
MS	–	80	90	100	–	110	114	120	130	20k
1	70	80	90	100	104	110	114	120	130	16k
2	70	80	90	100	104	110	114	120	130	12k
3	70	80	90	100	104	110	114	120	130	8k
1J	42	52	62	72	76	–	–	–	–	16k
2J	42	52	62	72	76	–	–	–	–	12k
3J	42	52	62	72	76	–	–	–	–	8k

Example ranking table

I recommend going online to find a federation in your country and checking out their website for specific rules and rankings. Even if you aren't competing in a competition, it is nice to know the rankings so you can create specific training goals.

PRIMARY DISCIPLINES

SNATCH

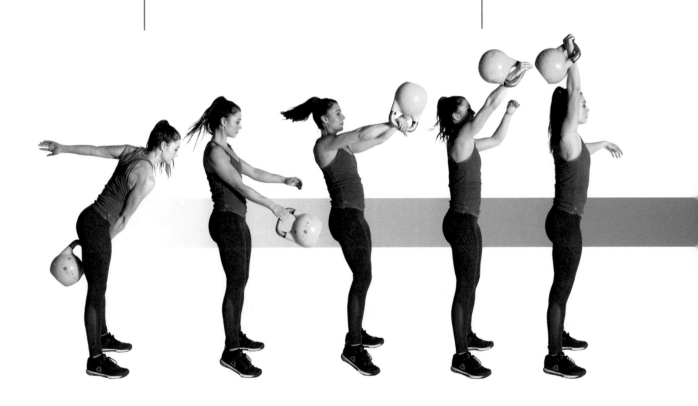

HALF SNATCH

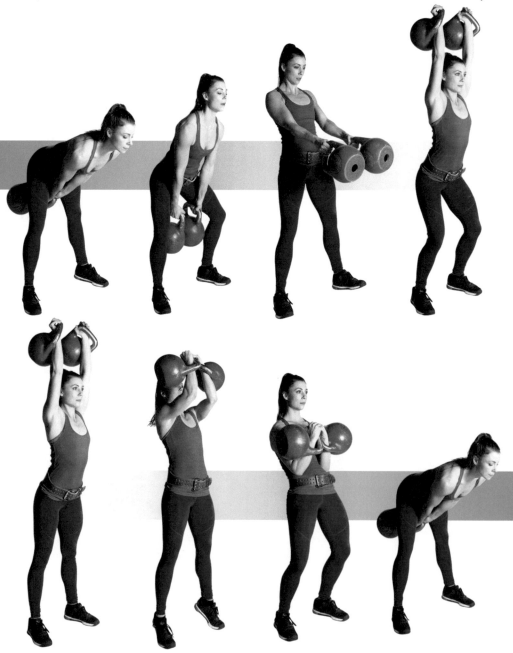

LONG CYCLE

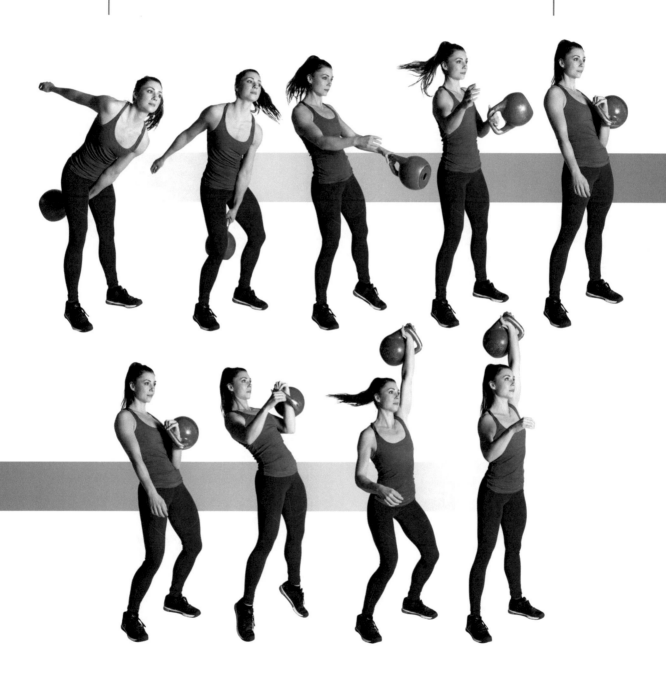

TWO-ARM LONG CYCLE

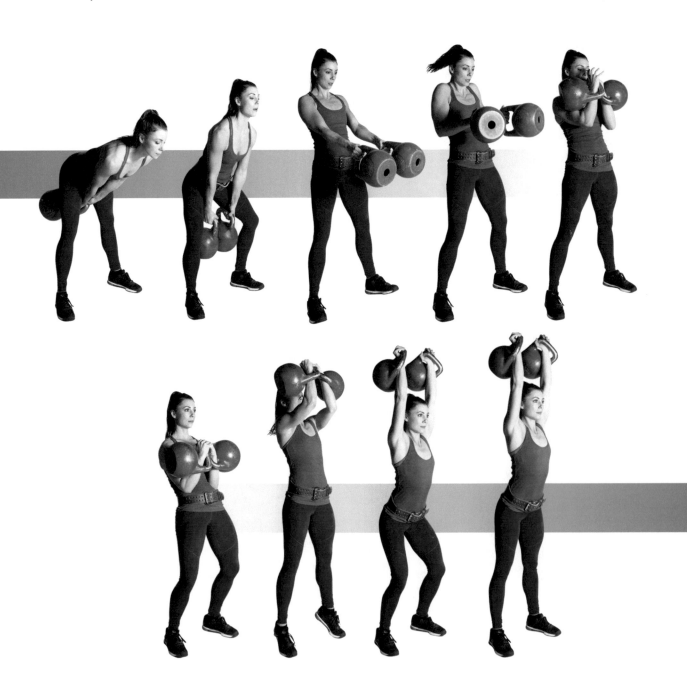

JERK

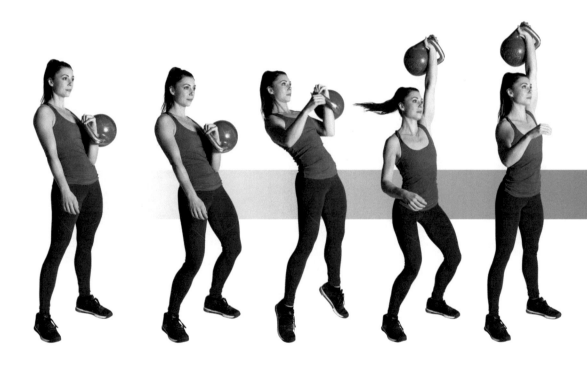

DOUBLE JERK

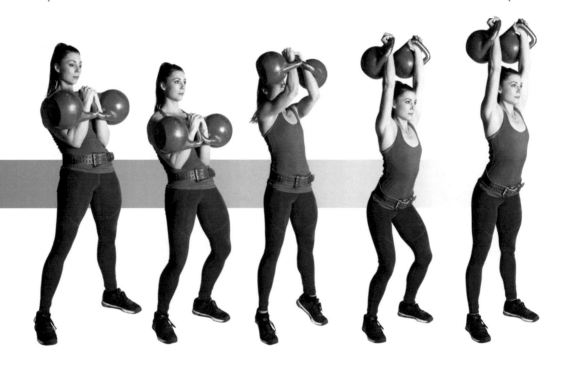

PENDULUM SWING

The pendulum or long swing is the primary type of swing used in kettlebell sport. The pendulum swing allows you to move the kettlebell using minimal effort while simultaneously creating as much momentum as possible. Devote time and attention to perfecting the pendulum swing, as it lays the foundation for a multitude of kettlebell movements. Consistent refinement of this technique not only maximizes efficiency in your workouts but also minimizes the risk of injury. The precision achieved through dedicated practice translates into improved coordination, stability, and power, unlocking the full potential of endurance based kettlebell training.

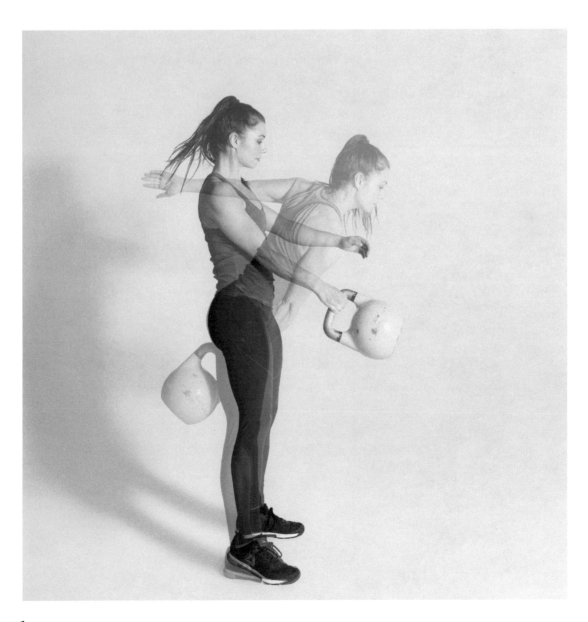

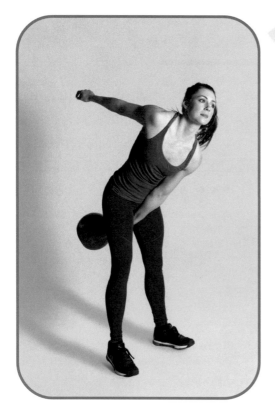

1.

Pull the arm "high and tight" between the legs.

Load the hamstrings by slightly straightening the legs. Loading the hamstrings allows the kettlebell to gain momentum by aiding in the creation of the pendulum motion.

Let the kettlebell reach the end of the pendulum and start to come forward on its own. Try not to aid the forward momentum of the pendulum by propelling or forcing it before it has started moving back between the legs on its own.

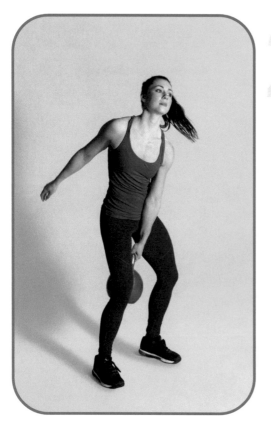

2.

Maintain a tall chest and bend the knees as the kettlebell starts to come forward.

Keep the arm tight to the body. Keeping the arm tight to the body allows you to successfully transfer the momentum of the pendulum along to the next phase of whatever lift you're performing.

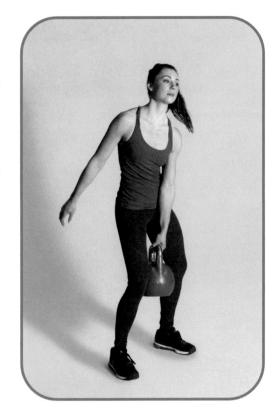

Squat slightly as the kettlebell transitions from behind the body to in front.

This is the point in the swing where you use the legs and glutes to power the forward motion of the bell by starting to stand up from that squat.

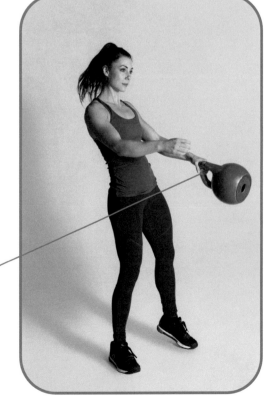

Stand up tall and lean back. This keeps the arm in contact with the body longer and keeps the kettlebell from pulling the shoulder unnecessarily.

Hold the kettlebell using a "Reverse Hook Grip".

Notice how the thumb sits on top of the finger

LOCKOUT/FIXATION

Lockout, or fixation, occurs in two places: in the overhead position and in the rack position. In the snatch exercise, there is only fixation once you've reached the overhead position. In jerks and long cycle, fixation occurs in both the rack and the overhead position after the jerk. In this section we'll go over the overhead and rack fixation requirements and tips for optimizing your efficiency.

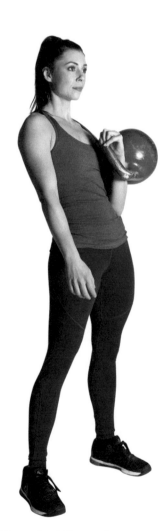

Rack Fixation

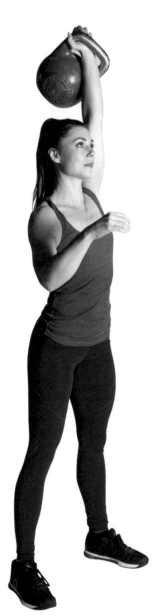

Overhead Fixation

Overhead lockout or fixation occurs when the kettlebell or kettlebells are overhead, the arm is straight, the knees and hips are open, and the kettlebells have stopped moving. Relaxing the forearms and hands and keeping the arms close to the ear are not mandatory, but will help you achieve the most energy-efficient position. This is a position you want to get comfortable being in so practice it diligently just like the pendulum swing.

OVERHEAD POSITION

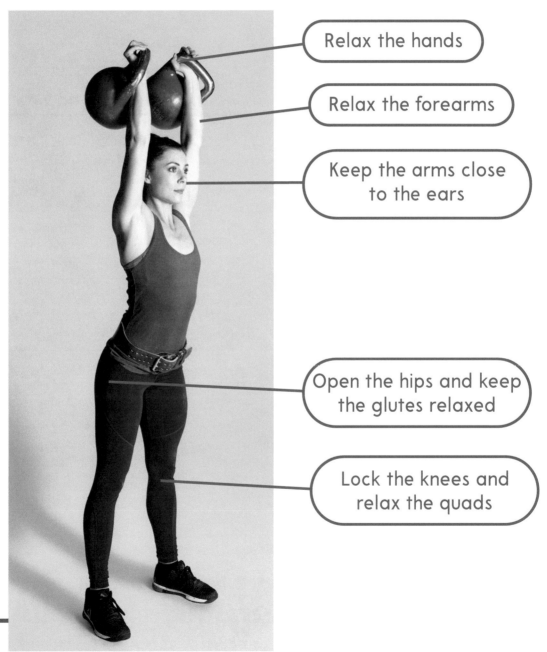

Relax the hands

Relax the forearms

Keep the arms close to the ears

Open the hips and keep the glutes relaxed

Lock the knees and relax the quads

The rack is where the kettlebells end up after the clean. It serves as a transition between the clean and jerk. It can also be one of the transition points for the double half snatch. Fixation in the rack position is a critical point in the lift to master. During competition, you'll need to show fixation in the rack position between reps for the rep to be considered valid. The rack is also considered a resting position for jerk and long cycle lifts.

RACK POSITION

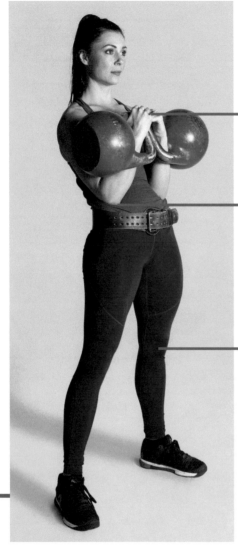

Relax the hands and forearms

If you're using two kettlebells, interlock handles to maximize their stability

Keep elbows tight to body

Support the elbow on the hip's iliac crest. If your elbow is unable to reach the hip, keep them tight to the torso to maximize the transfer of momentum from the legs

Lock the knees

Knees must completely straighten before the jerk occurs for the rep to be counted as valid

IF THE OVERHEAD LOCKOUT OR RACK POSITION IS DIFFICULT TO ACHIEVE, WORK ON SHOULDER AND THORACIC MOBILITY BEFORE AND AFTER EACH TRAINING SESSION. FIND THE BEST POSITION FOR YOUR BODY TYPE. YOU SHOULD NOT FEEL ANY PINCHING IN THE LOW BACK.

SNATCH

The snatch is when the kettlebell travels from between the legs to the overhead position in one continuous motion. The rep is completed when you've achieved lockout/fixation of the arm, shoulder, hips and knees.

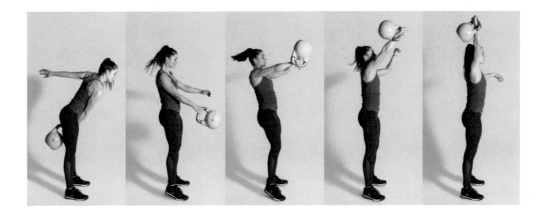

Tips

Breathe Methodically (timed breathing). There are breathing techniques specific to each movement that are typically used once some of the other basics are mastered. When you're first learning, it's most important to just breathe for all the sport movements.

Be Patient. Wait for the kettlebell to come back on its own from the back swing and wait for it to be weightless before initiating the pull.

Initiate the "cast" or "drop" by rotating the hand outwards - lean back and let the bell fall instead of throwing the shoulder forward to initiate the descent of the kettlebell.

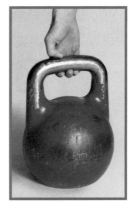

FINGERTIP GRIP

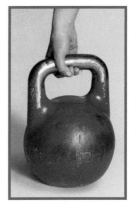

REVERSE HOOK GRIP

Cast/drop = the section of the movement when the bell is brought from overhead/rack position back down to the swing for the next rep.

SNATCH BASICS

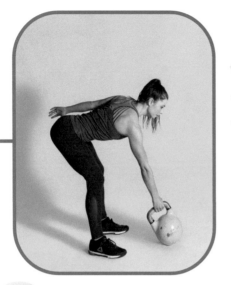

1. When you pull the kettlebell off of the floor for the first swing or snatch, send the hips back, keep your back flat, and pull the kettlebell high between the legs. This is the ideal starting position for all sport lifts.

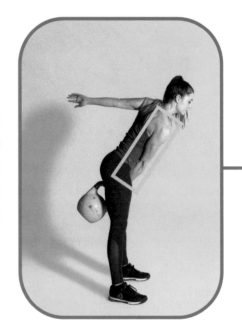

2. Notice the position of the arm. Keep the arm high and tight throughout the entire swing. Failure to sustain the arm position can lead to the kettlebell dropping too low between the legs, resulting in premature disconnection of the arm and reduced momentum transfer.

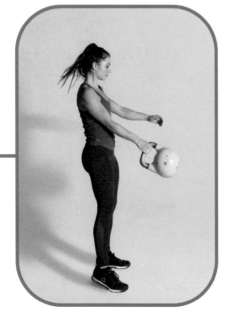

3. When the bell starts its way back forward, drive off the opposite leg and keep the arm connected to your body until you've reached full/triple extension.*

This is also the point where the kettlebell becomes weightless. Here, you retract the shoulder to change the trajectory of the kettlebell from forward to up.

*Full or triple extension occurs when the hip, knee and ankle have all fully extended. Ankle extension amount will vary based on the weight and technique.

4. Start to open the hand here to begin the insertion phase of the lift. This is when the hand shifts from the swinging phase of the lift to the catch position.

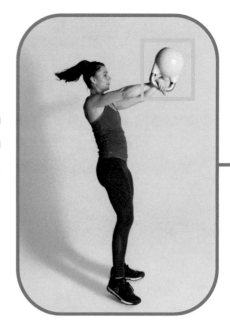

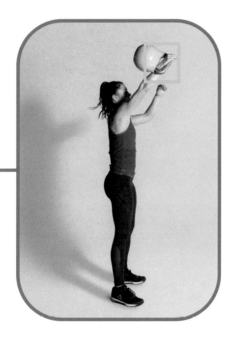

5. The hand should be completely inserted by this point. The momentum of the kettlebell will bring the arm by the ear.

6. The center mass of the kettlebell should be over your body's center of mass to create maximum stability.

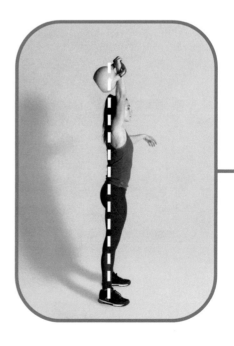

INSERTING THE HAND TOO LATE OR HAVING TOO TIGHT OF A GRIP ON THE HANDLE CAN CAUSE THE BELL TO BANG THE ARM AND/OR PULL THE SHOULDER TOO FAR BACK IN THE OVERHEAD POSITION.

SNATCH PHASES

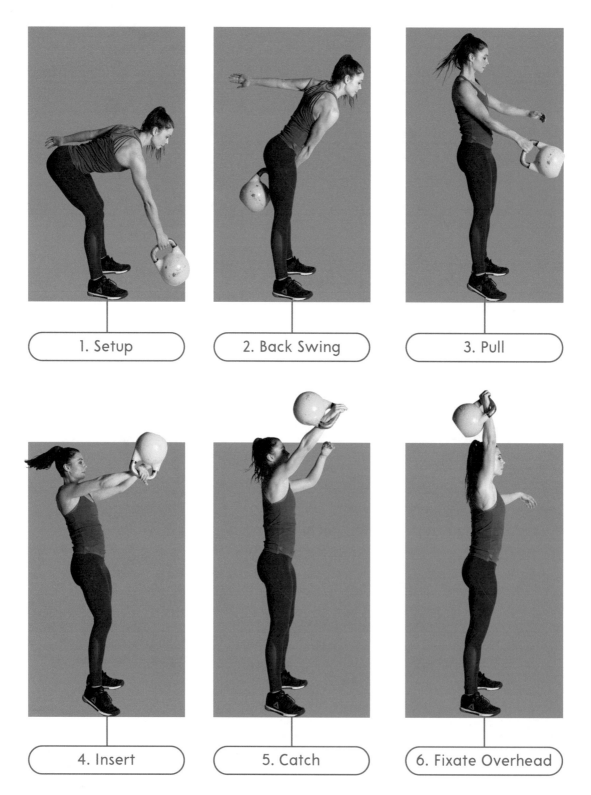

1. Setup

2. Back Swing

3. Pull

4. Insert

5. Catch

6. Fixate Overhead

SNATCH PHASES

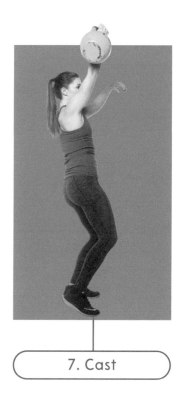

7. Cast

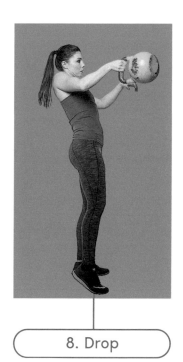

8. Drop

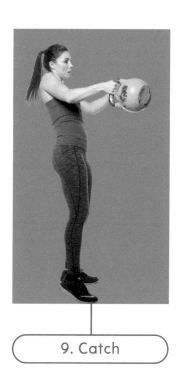

9. Catch

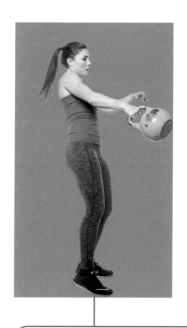

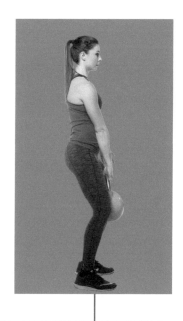

10. Absorption

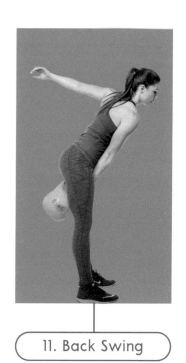

11. Back Swing

JERK

The jerk begins with the kettlebell in the rack position. The legs bend slightly ("first dip"), and as the legs are powerfully straightened ("bump"), the kettlebell is pressed to a lockout position and caught in a quarter squat ("second dip"). The legs and hips fully extend as you hold the lockout position. The rep is complete when you've achieved lockout/fixation of the arm, shoulder, hips and knees.

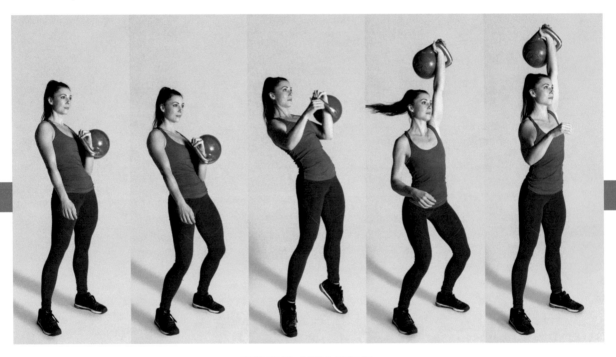

SINGLE-ARM JERK

Tips

Keep the arm and elbow tight to the body in the rack and first dip. Be quick and explosive. Do not pause during the first dip.

Keep the elbow connected as you drive or bump the kettlebell from the hip or chest.

Depending on your body type, the arm will sit high on the chest or low on the hip.

Stabilize the kettlebells before standing up from the second dip.

JERK BASICS

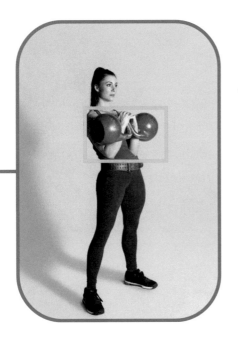

1. Interlock the hands or kettlebell handles and keep the elbows tight to the body for maximum stability. If aligning the handles directly on top of one another proves challenging, ensure that, at the very least, the handles remain in contact with each other.

2. Maintain a neutral spine as you dip into the knees. This knee dip will help keep the elbows close to the body, facilitating the maximum transfer of momentum. Dipping into the knees will ensure that the kettlebells track in a straighter line. Remember not to pause in the bottom of this position; you should be quick and explosive.

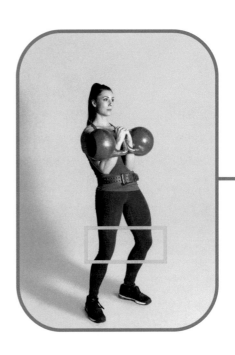

Place one hand over the other. Do not interlock the fingers.

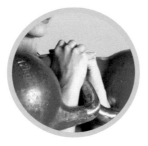

AVOID SENDING THE BUTT BACK ON THE FIRST DIP, THIS WILL CAUSE THE ELBOWS TO DISCONNECT EARLY OR THE TORSO TO DROP TOO FAR FORWARD.

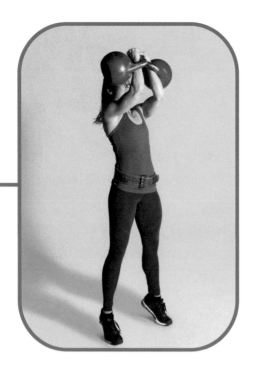

3. Drive the elbows off of the hips.

Be sure to achieve triple extension before dropping under the kettlebells.

4. Catch the bells in a stance where your hips are pushed back, and your weight rests on your heels. Stabilize the bells in this position before standing up.

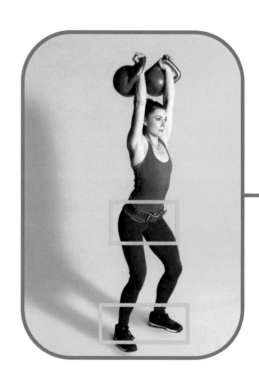

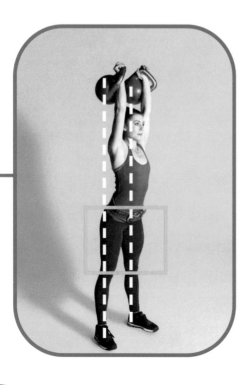

5. Stand up and keep the quads relaxed. The center of mass of the kettlebells should be over your body's center mass. To maintain a more relaxed stance upon standing, remind yourself to push your knees back for leg straightening rather than pushing the hips forward.

JERK PHASES

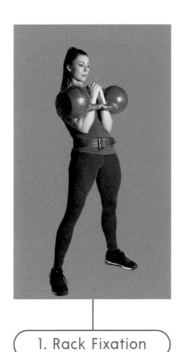

1. Rack Fixation

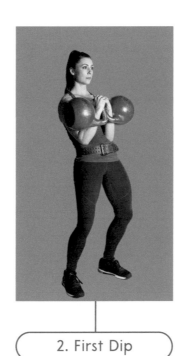

2. First Dip

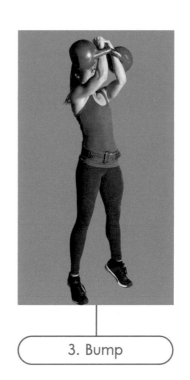

3. Bump

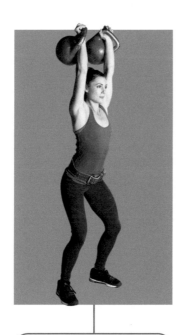

4. Second Dip

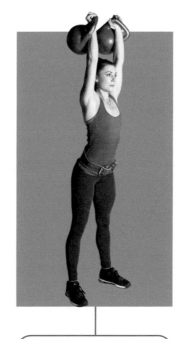

5. Overhead Fixation

JERK PHASES

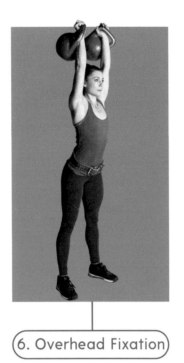

6. Overhead Fixation

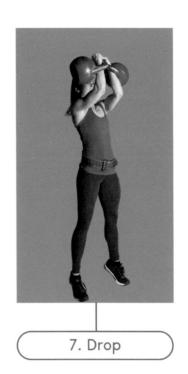

7. Drop

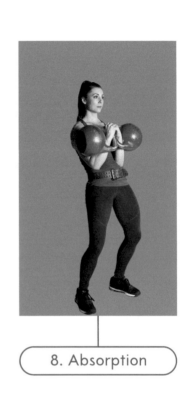

8. Absorption

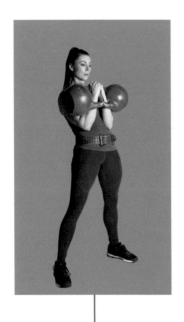

9. Rack Fixation

When transitioning from the overhead fixated position to the rack position, allow the kettlebells to drop freely in front of your shoulders while simultaneously bending your legs to absorb the weight. Then, stabilize yourself in the rack position by straightening your legs.

It's important not to exert unnecessary control over the kettlebells during their descent, as this will add extra, unneeded effort

CLEAN

The clean is when you swing the kettlebell between the legs into the rack position in one continuous motion. The rep is complete when the kettlebell has fixated in the rack and the hips and knees are locked.

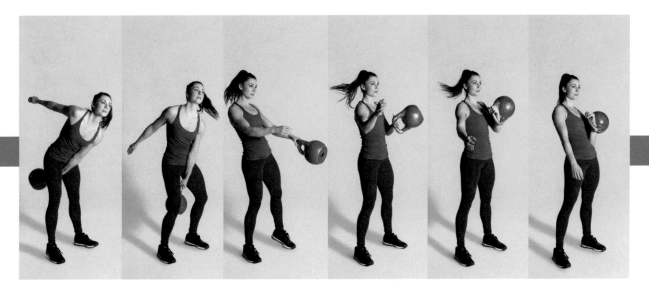

SINGLE-ARM CLEAN

Tips

Keep the arms tight to the body for the entire movement.

Drive back onto the heels and only pull the weight towards your body once the kettlebells have reached a weightless point.

Work on achieving hand insertion as early as possible.

Initiate the "cast" or "drop" by rotating the hands and letting the bells fall. Do not throw the shoulders forward to initiate the cast/drop.

CLEAN BASICS

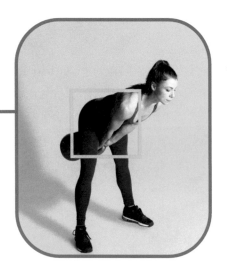

1. Keep the arms tight to the torso, hands up high between the legs, and load the hamstrings at the back of the swing.

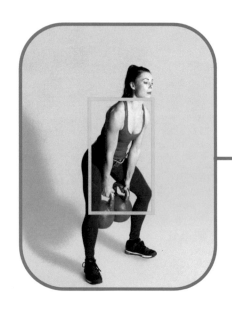

2. Keep the shoulders seated and arms connected to the torso until the torso is perpendicular to the floor.

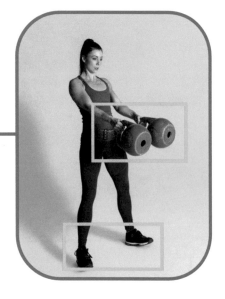

3. Drive back on to the heels or achieve triple extension in this phase of the lift.

Be patient and wait for the bells to reach a weightless or floating state before initiating the pull.

4. Initiate the pull by bringing the elbows in and shrugging the shoulders simultaneously.

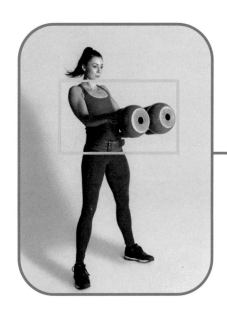

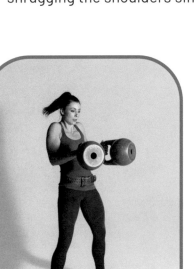

5. Insert the hands once the kettlebells feel weightless.

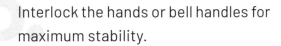

6. Interlock the hands or bell handles for maximum stability.

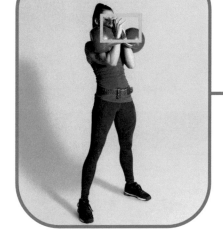

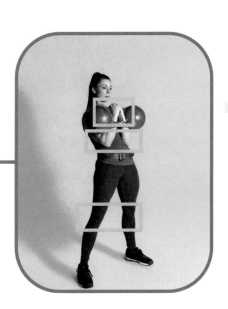

7. Keep hands interlocked or bells interlocked, keep elbows in tight, straighten the legs and relax the quads.

CLEAN PHASES

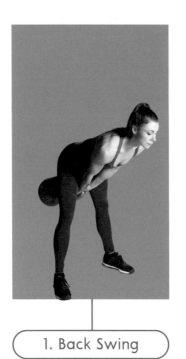

1. Back Swing

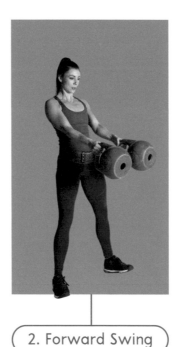

2. Forward Swing

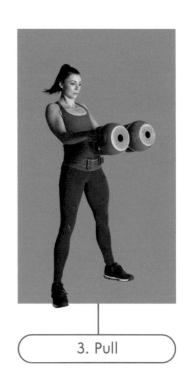

3. Pull

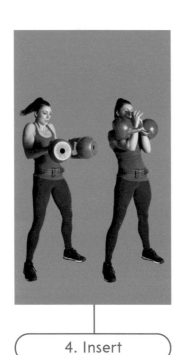

4. Insert

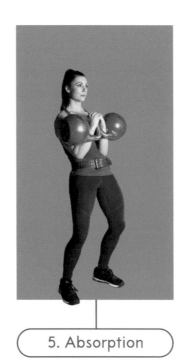

5. Absorption

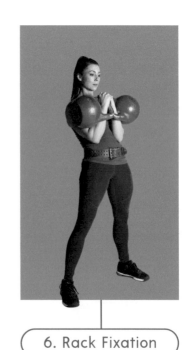

6. Rack Fixation

FITNESS OUTSIDE THE BOX

LONG CYCLE

Long cycle (AKA clean and jerk) is when you swing the kettlebell between the legs and into the rack position, show rack fixation, and then perform a jerk. The rep is complete when the kettlebell has fixated overhead.

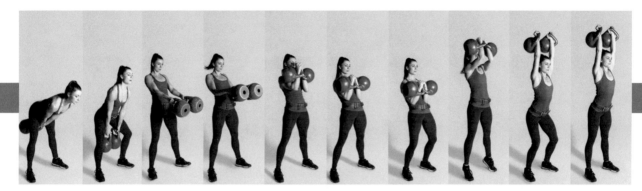

TWO-ARM LONG CYCLE

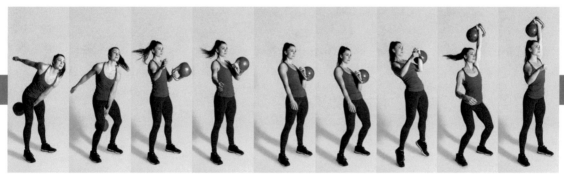

SINGLE-ARM LONG CYCLE

—— Tips

Follow the same principles of the clean and jerk as shown previously.

Be sure to pause between the clean and jerk phases.

After completing the clean and jerk, bring the arms straight down through the rack and right into the next clean. In other words, do not pause in the rack after performing the jerk.

HALF SNATCH

Half snatch is when you bring one or two kettlebells from between the legs to overhead in one continuous motion. The rep is complete when you have achieved lockout/fixation of the arm, shoulder, hips and knees. The kettlebells are then brought down through the rack position before you complete the next rep.

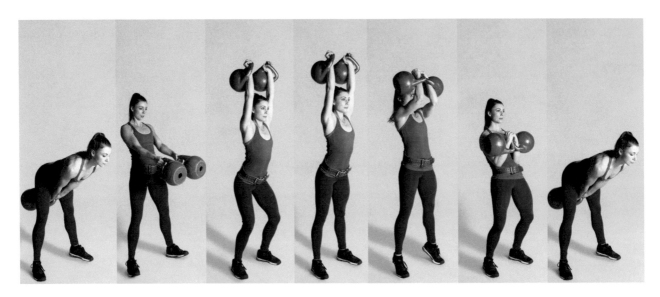

DOUBLE HALF SNATCH

Tips

Follow the same principles of the snatch and jerk as shown previously.

As soon as the bells are weightless, initiate the pull by retracting the shoulders and drop under the weight, similar to the second dip of the jerk. Once the bells are stable, stand up and establish fixation.

On the way down, drop the bells through the rack, absorb the weight with the legs, and drop into the next swing. Keep the arms high and tight to the body during the swing.

SPORT HAND POSITIONS

SPORT GRIP

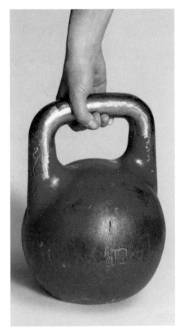

The reverse hook grip, recognized as the optimal grip for kettlebell sport movements, not only provides a secure hold but also affords the advantage of an open hand, facilitating seamless transitions between the swing and insertion phases of the lifts. Mastering this grip technique will significantly enhance your performance.

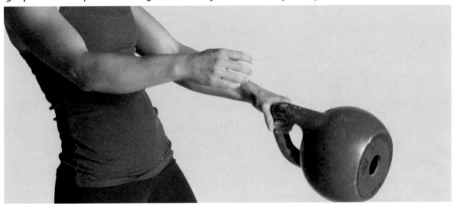

OVERHEAD

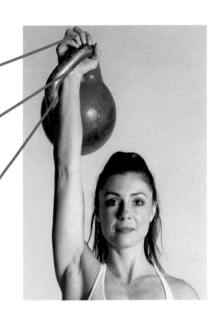

Relax the fingers

Support majority of the bell weight on the ulna

Let the bell rest on the arm; try to eliminate space between the bell and the arm

TIPS FOR SUCCESS IN KETTLEBELL SPORT

1) Master the Technique

Success in kettlebell sport requires performing each lift with proper technique which requires consistency, dedication, and constant analysis. It's imperative that you spend time perfecting your form and mastering the technique of each lift. Mastering the technique will help you lift efficiently, reduce your risk of injury, and maximize your performance. Perfect practice makes perfect.

2) Build Endurance and Strength

Kettlebell sport requires both endurance and strength. Train exercises that focus on building your cardiovascular endurance, such as running, rowing, biking or swimming, along with strength training exercises like, deadlifts, squats, presses and rows. A strong foundation and a balance of endurance and strength will help achieve a high level of performance during kettlebell sets. Only training the sport movements is not enough to keep the body balanced and in optimal shape.

3) Routinely Practice

Consistency is key to success. Create a training plan and stick to it. Commit to practicing regularly and progressively increase your training volume and workload over time. Progressively increasing will build your stamina, strength and technique. It is essential to listen to your body! Take rest days when needed, or restructure your training to avoid overtraining. Consistency isn't just about maintaining the same intensity but also adapting your plan to your evolving fitness levels and goals.

4) Prepare Mentally

Kettlebell sport is physically demanding and mentally challenging. Visualize yourself performing well during training sessions and competitions. Practice positive self-talk to build confidence. Success isn't just about how much you can lift; it's also about maintaining a strong mindset.

5) Train with Awareness

Pay attention to the intensity of your training. Gradually increase the weight, sets and reps in your training. Monitor and track your progress. Avoid pushing yourself too hard too quickly. Progressing faster than your body is ready for can result in burnout or injury. It's always a good idea to consider working with a qualified coach who can provide guidance and feedback on your technique. A knowledgeable coach can offer personalized insights, helping you navigate the intricacies of periodization and tailoring your program to align with your individual fitness aspirations.

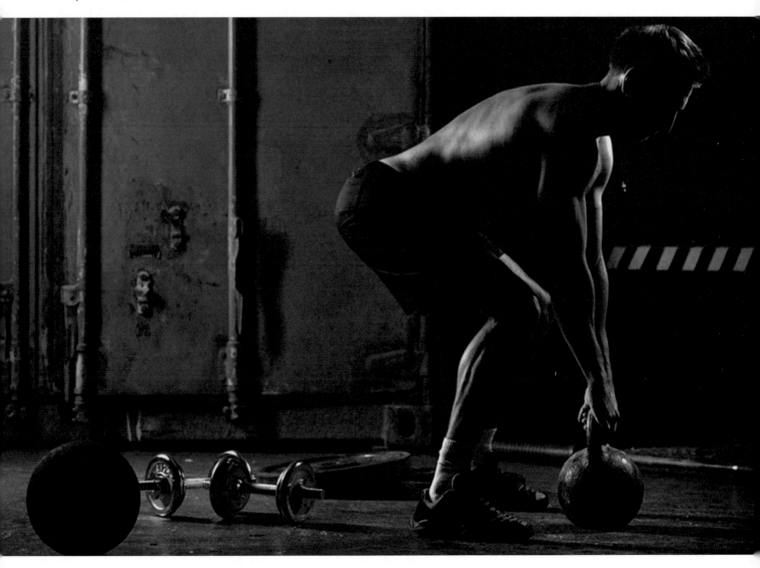

Achieving success in kettlebell sport demands dedication, ongoing practice, and considerable patience. Enhance your performance and attain your goals by emphasizing technique, enhancing endurance and strength, staying attuned to your body, and cultivating mental tenacity.

MOVEMENTS

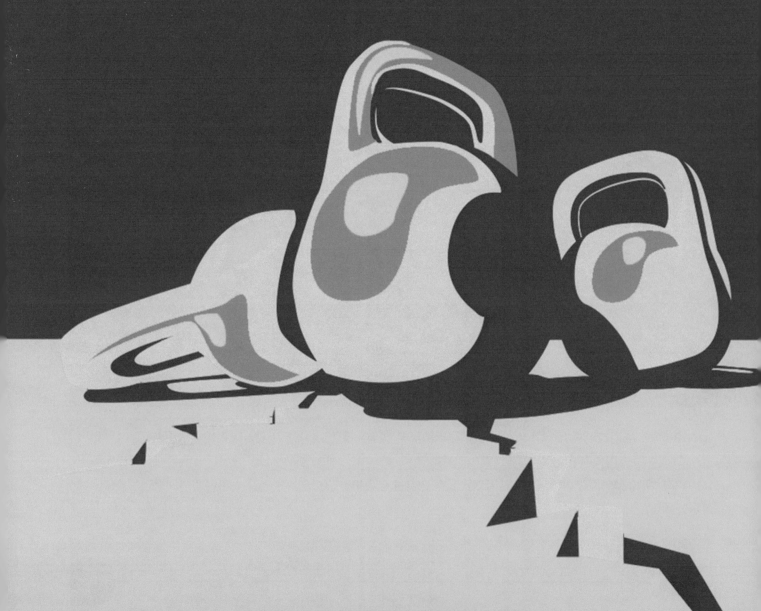

GRIPS & RACKS

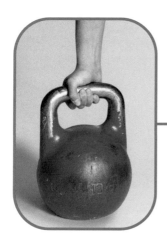

TIGHT GRIP
Used for exercises where maximum forearm engagement is desired

FINGER GRIP (Monkey Grip)
Can be used for exercises when the goal is to strengthen the fingers

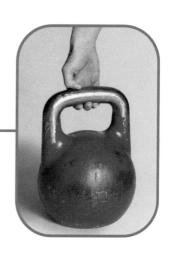

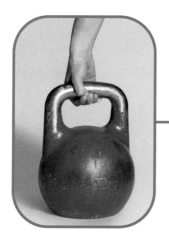

HOOK GRIP
Used for maximum gripping capabilities with minimal forearm engagement (thumb under fingers)

REVERSE HOOK GRIP
This hybrid fingertip grip and hook grip is best used for sport movements

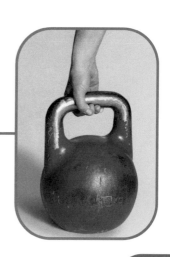

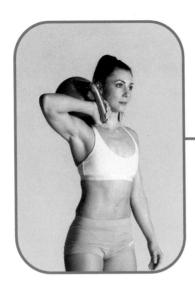

POTATO SACK RACK

Best used for the exercises where you want less shoulder activation

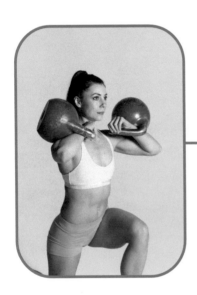

FITNESS RACK

Best used for general exercises or when potato sack rack is not comfortable

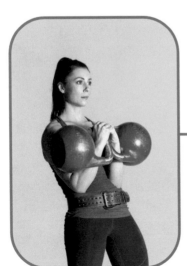

SPORT RACK

Best used for sport movements

HOLDS

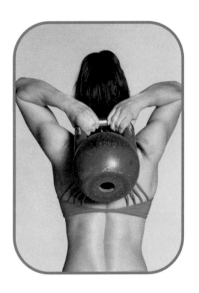

BEHIND THE NECK

Kettlebell rests on upper back

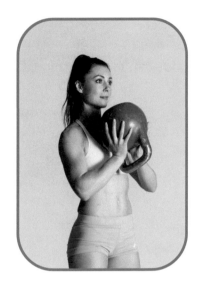

GOBLET

Kettlebell is supported by palms of hands and chest

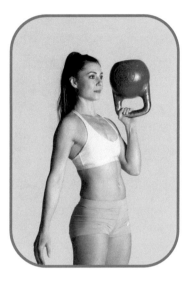

BOTTOMS UP

Kettlebell is supported by palm - must use a tight grip

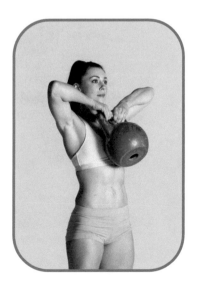

TWO HAND

Both hands grip the kettlebell equally

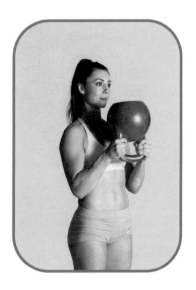

NEUTRAL

Hands are grabbing the "horns" of the kettlebell

BODY POSITION BASICS

Exactly how we move during an exercise is somewhat dependent on the exercise itself. But there are a few keys I find helpful to think about across the majority of movements. Focusing on these cues offers a comprehensive approach to movement, ensuring successful execution and maximizing the benefits of a wide range of exercises.

These are the cues I most commonly use before and during the exercise:

- Tall/High Chest
- Shoulders Down and Back
- Neutral Spine (including your neck)

- Active Legs
- Active Core

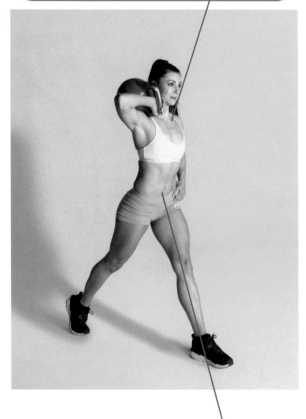

Maintain a flat back

Think about keeping your chest high and the shoulders seated (down and back)

Keep the legs active by sitting back into the glutes and slightly drive the knee outward

Pull the belly in slightly to activate the core

LOWER BODY EXERCISES

DEADLIFTS (DL)

Perform the deadlift by placing the feet underneath the hips. You might use a narrow or wide stance depending on the style of deadlift you're doing. Send the hips and butt back while keeping your chest high. Maintain tension in this position as you pick up the weight. Think about lifting the weight with your chest and legs versus lifting with your back. Drive the knees out, keep the back flat, and pull the stomach in.

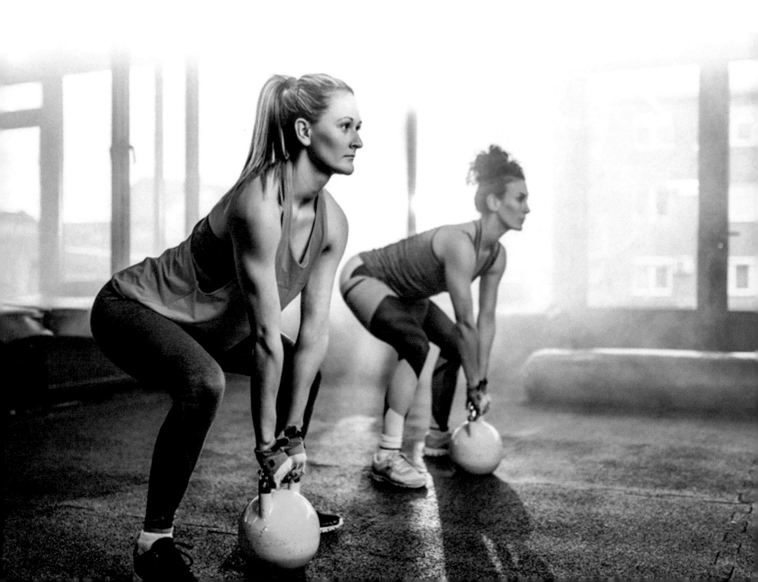

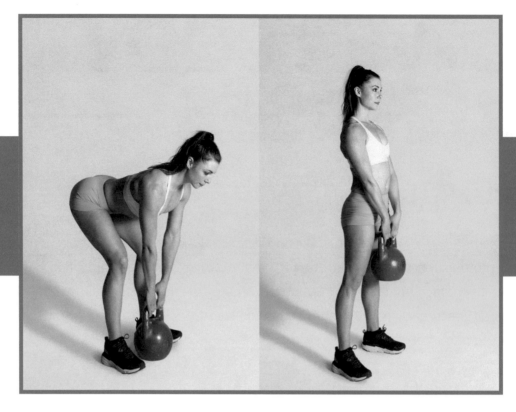

Conventional DL - 1 KB

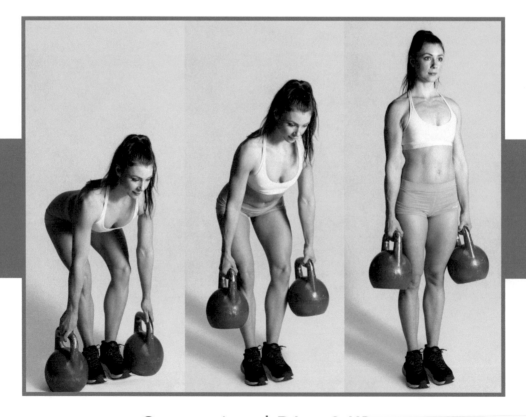

Conventional DL - 2 KB

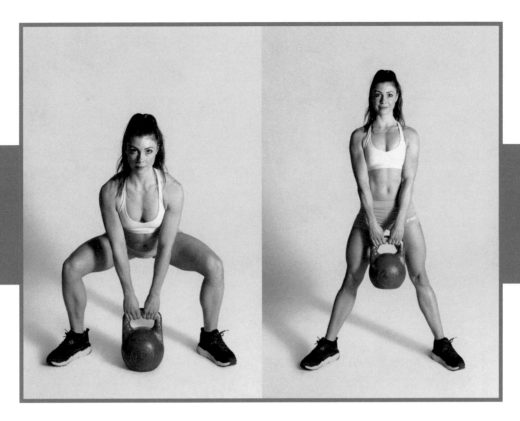

Sumo DL - 1 KB

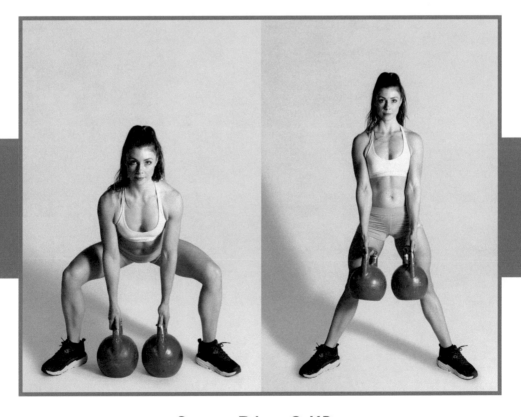

Sumo DL - 2 KB

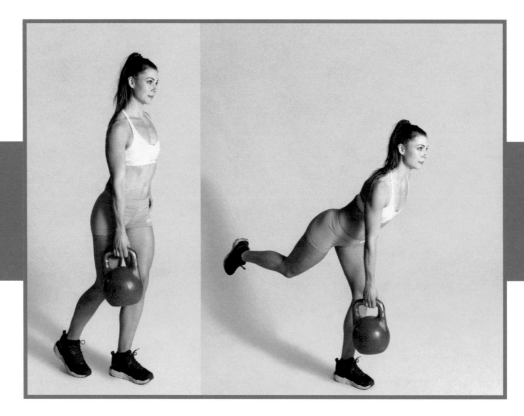

Single-Leg DL - 1 KB

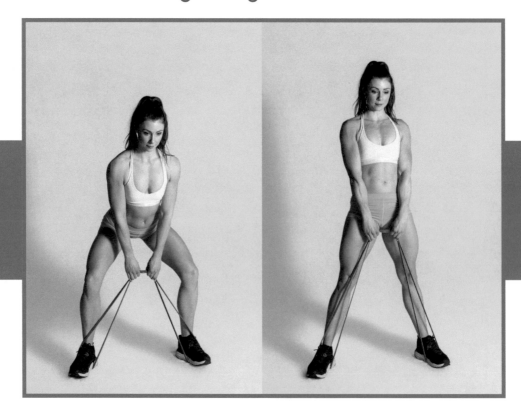

Banded DL

SQUATS

To set up for most styles of squats, place your feet just outside the hips. How wide apart they are will vary depending on which type of squat you're performing.

The feet can be pointed straight or slightly turned out. Send your butt back first to initiate the squat, then bend the knees. Sending the butt back will shift the weight to the heels. Press the knees slightly out as you squat to keep the hips and knees stable during the movement.

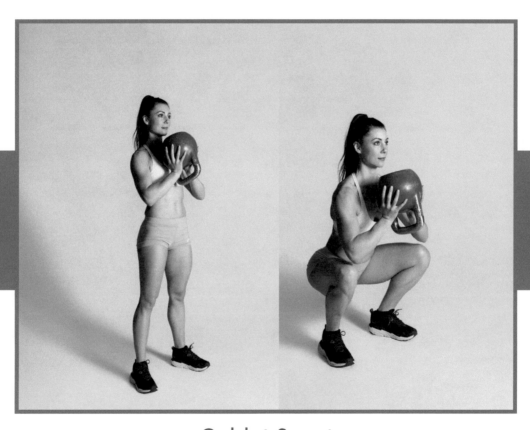

Goblet Squat

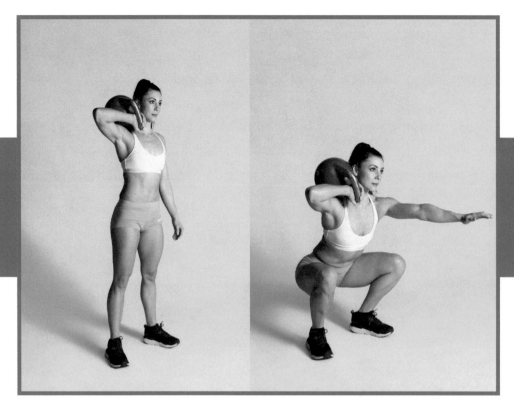

Squat (potato sack rack)

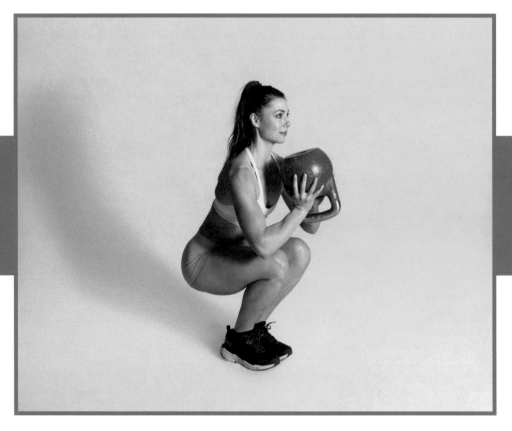

Narrow Stance Squat

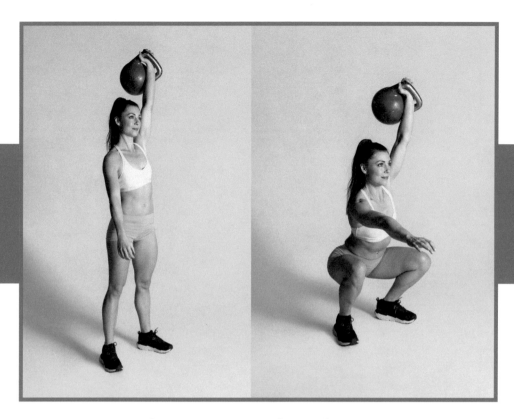

Single-Arm Overhead Squat

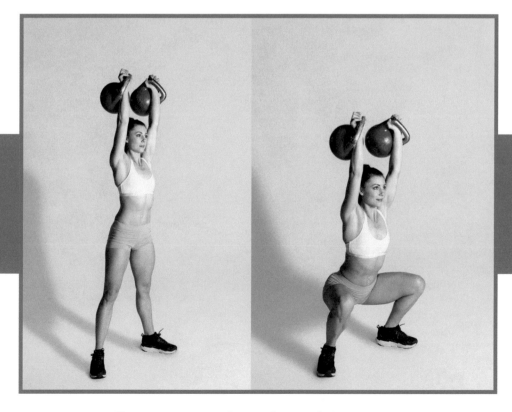

Two-Arm Overhead Squat

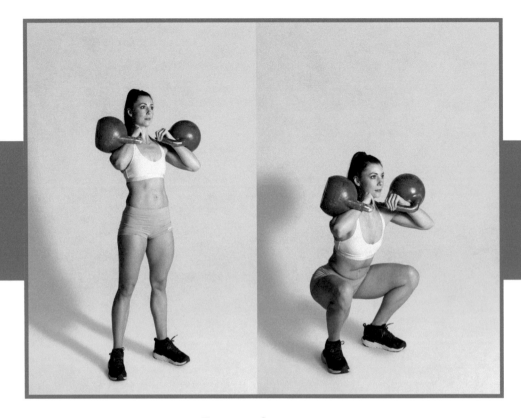

Front Squat

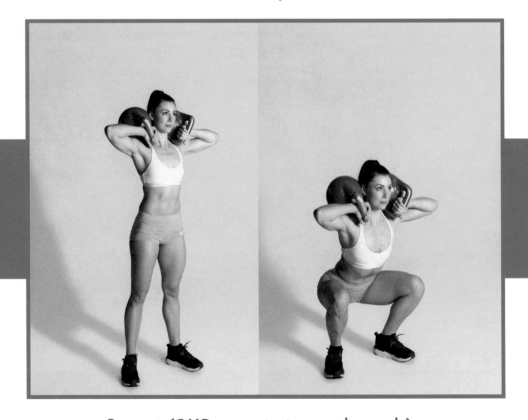

Squat (2KB - potato sack rack)

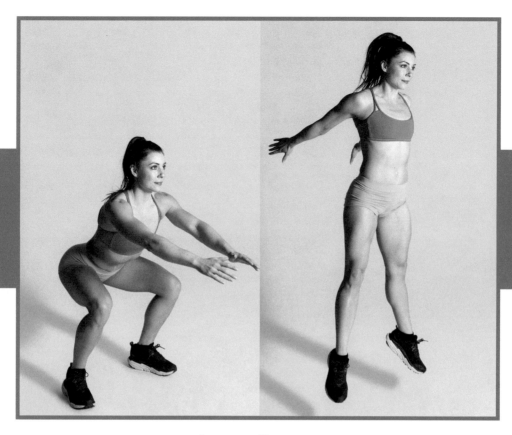

Jump Squat

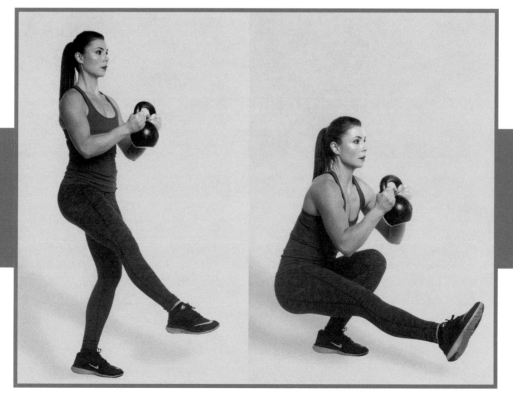

Single-Leg Squat (pistol squat)

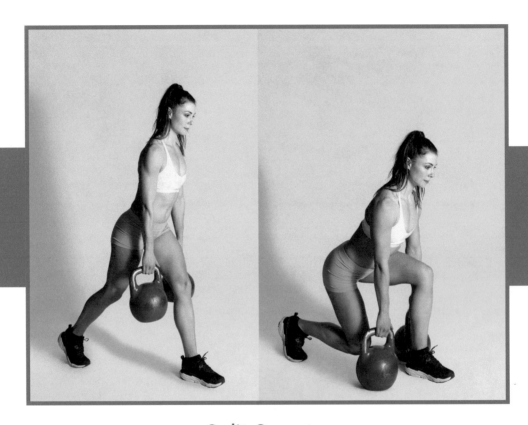

Split Squat

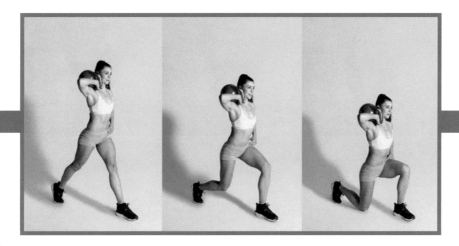

Split Squat Variation

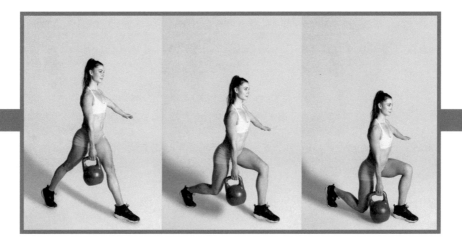

Split Squat Variation

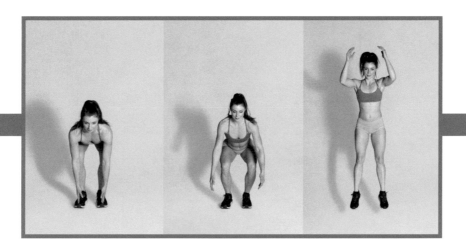

Jump Squat Variation

LUNGES

To activate more of the hamstring (back of leg) and the glute (buttock) during lunges and single-leg movements, keep the shin as vertical as possible and shift the weight onto the heel of the front foot. You can also think about pressing the knee outward to activate those posterior muscles and create additional stability.

To activate more of the quadriceps (front of leg), lunge with the knee over the toes.

Pay attention to how your weight distribution between feet changes what muscles are activated.

Keep a tall chest and pull your belly in to maintain a tight core and protect the back. Squeezing the shoulder blades together can help get your chest in the ideal position.

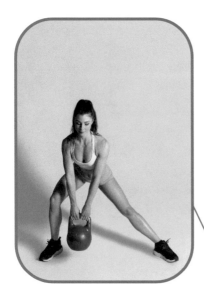

SIDE LUNGE

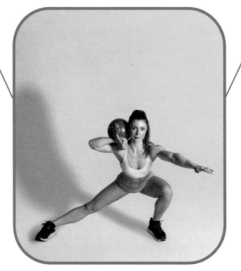

COSSACK LUNGE

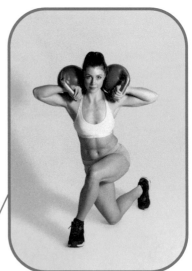

CURTSY LUNGE

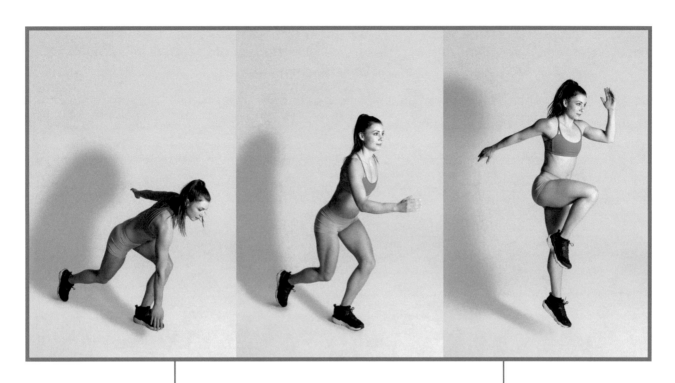

RUNNER'S LUNGE

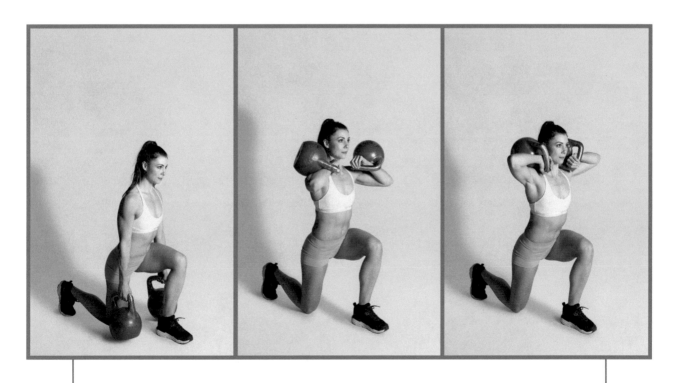

LUNGES WITH VARIOUS RACK POSITIONS

LOWER BODY FOCUSED CARDIO

Ensure systematic breathing during the exercise, directing your focus to exhaling deliberately during the explosive phase (exertion). The inhalation process will occur instinctively. Additionally, emphasize the importance of being light on your feet when landing from jumps—absorb the shock by gently bending the knees, promoting joint health and overall stability.

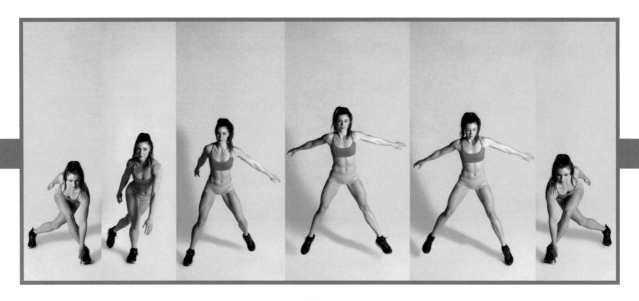

SKATER

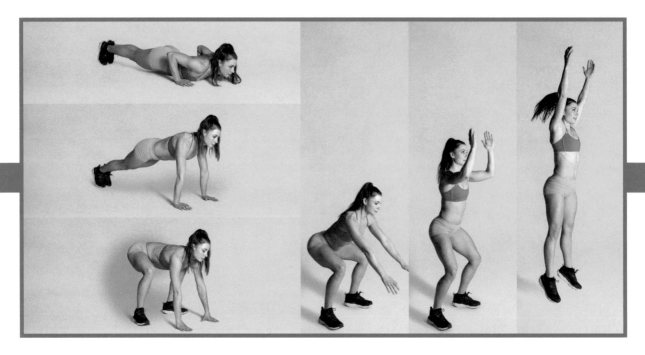

BURPEE

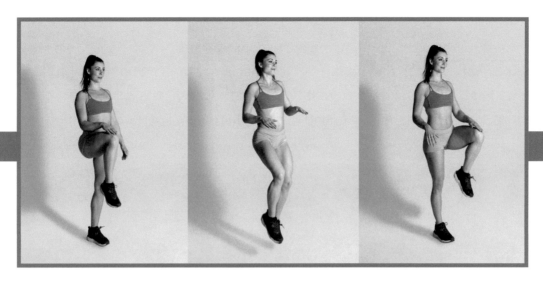

HIGH KNEES

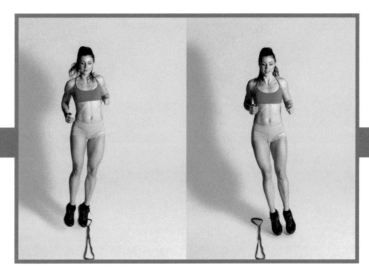

LATERAL HOPS

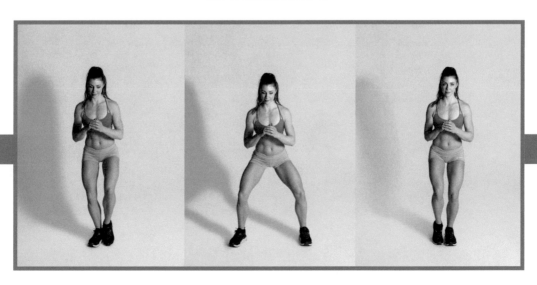

SIDE SHUFFLE

Perform the thruster in one continuous movement upwards (don't pause between the squat and press). Think about driving up through the heels or standing up hard. You can also think about thrusting the hips forward so that the glute activation is explosive. This will make the weight fly up, and the arms will only need to assist in the final part of the arm extension.

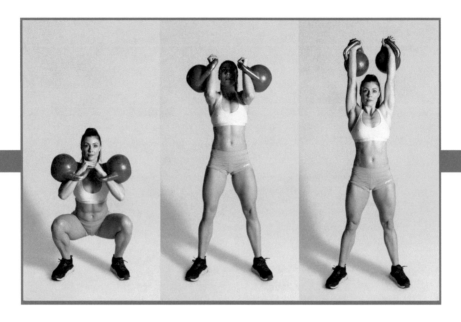

TWO-ARM THRUSTER

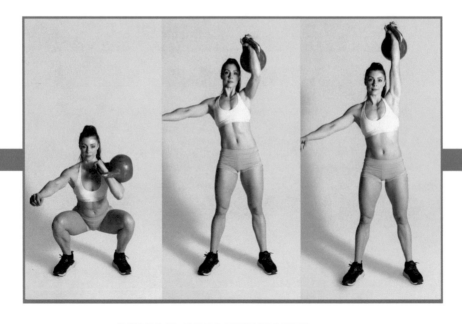

SINGLE-ARM THRUSTER

ADDITIONAL LOWER BODY

Focus your thoughts on the body part you're targeting. Keep your attention on that body part as you move through the exercise. There are also some physical things you can do to keep your attention on the body part. For example, when working your glutes squeeze your butt at the top of each rep. When performing leg extensions or squats, give your quads a good squeeze once you've straightened your legs.

On the Good Morning exercise, feel a good stretch in your hamstrings and maintain a tall chest while keeping your belly pulled in.

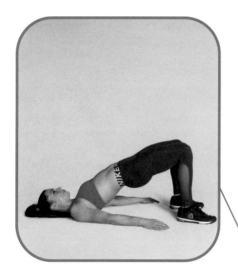

GLUTE BRIDGE

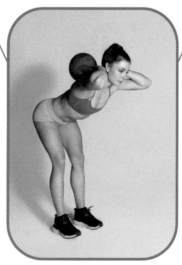

GOOD MORNING

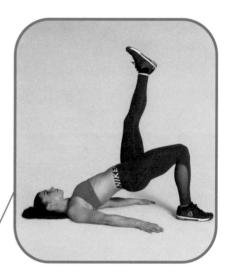

SINGLE-LEG GLUTE BRIDGE

KETTLEBELL SPORT & FITNESS BASICS

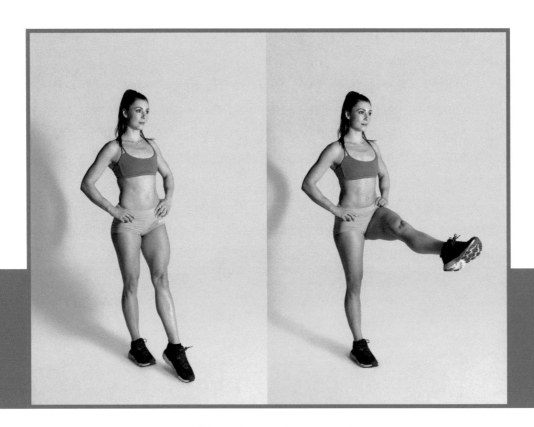

Standing Leg Extension

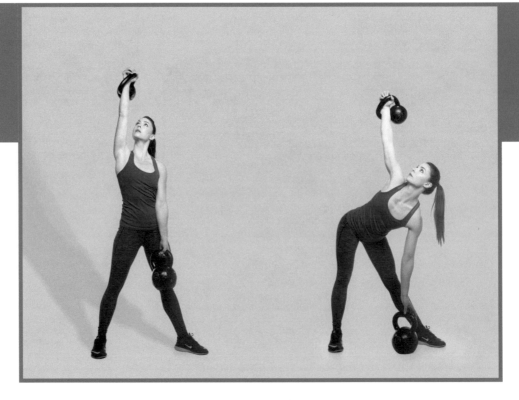

Windmill

UPPER BODY & ABDOMINAL EXERCISES

Prior to beginning most back exercises, set the shoulders by rolling the shoulders down and back and squeezing the shoulder blades together. Maintain that seated shoulder (down-and-back) position as you move through the reps.

Control the eccentric phase of the movement by not letting the weight or band tug the arm or shoulder uncontrollably. The eccentric phase of an exercise occurs when the muscles lengthen under load. An example of this would be the second part of the bicep curl - the part of the lift when the arm or weight is moving towards the floor.

Maintain an athletic stance by keeping the back flat, the chest tall, and the knees and hips slightly externally rotated. Externally rotating the knees and hips creates stability in the hip and knee joints. You can think about driving your knees out just a little or spreading the floor apart with your feet.

BACK

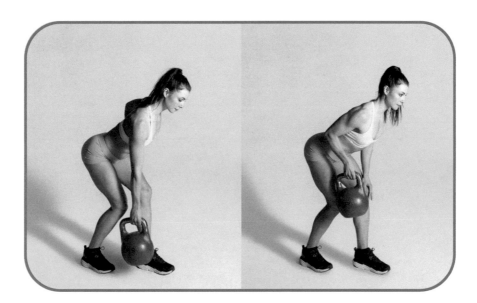

Single-Arm Row

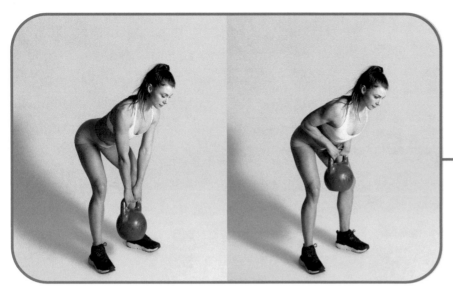

Narrow Grip Row

Two-Arm Row

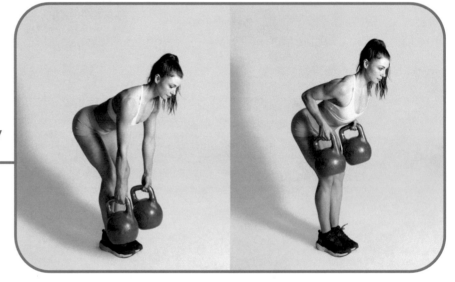

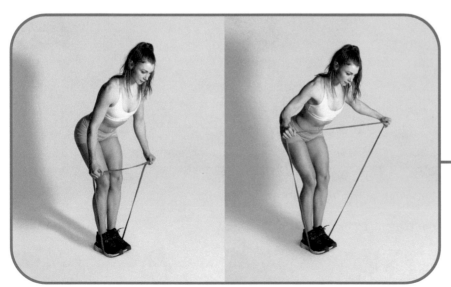

Banded
Reverse Fly

Renegade Row

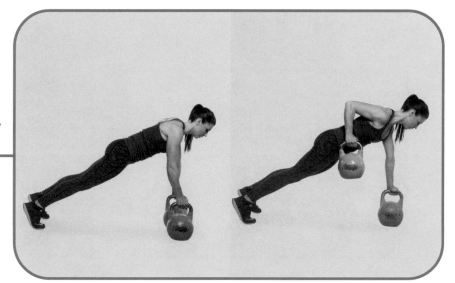

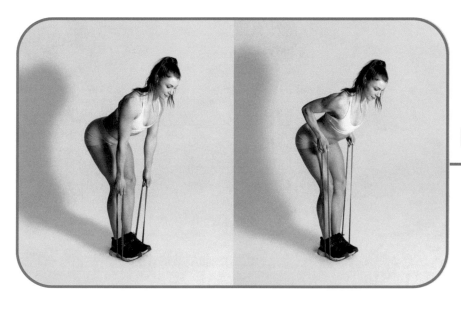

Banded Row

Band Pull-Apart

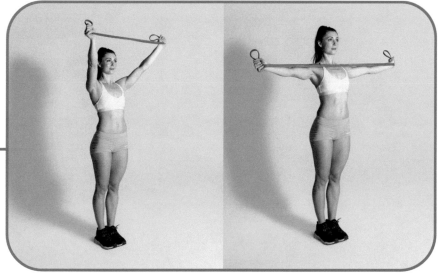

BICEPS & TRICEPS

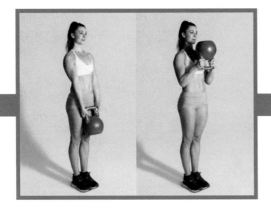

KB Curl

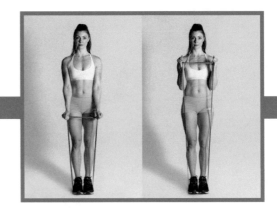

Neutral Grip Hammer Curl

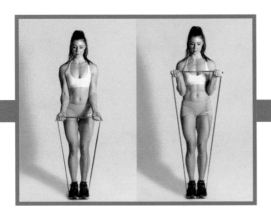

Banded Curl

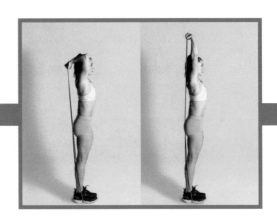

Two-Arm Overhead
Tricep Extension

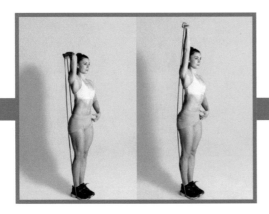

Single-Arm Overhead
Tricep Extension

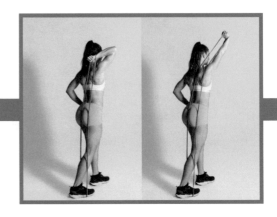

Single-Arm Tricep
Extension Variation

Maximize muscle contraction by squeezing the biceps or triceps at the end of each rep, focusing on maintaining a controlled and deliberate movement throughout the entire range of motion for optimal results.

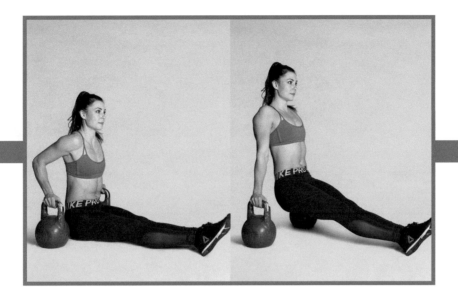

Dip

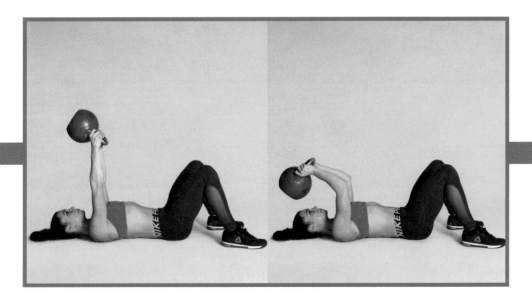

Skull Crusher

CHEST & SHOULDERS

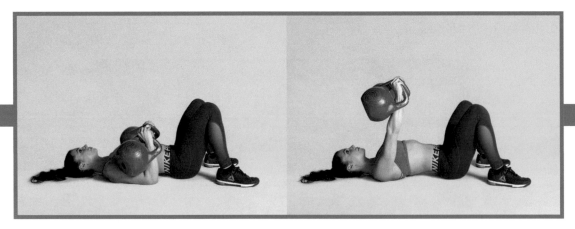

Chest or Floor Press

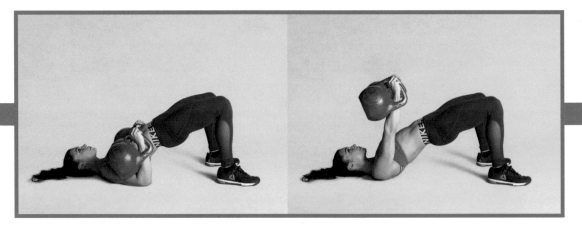

Hip Bridge Chest Press

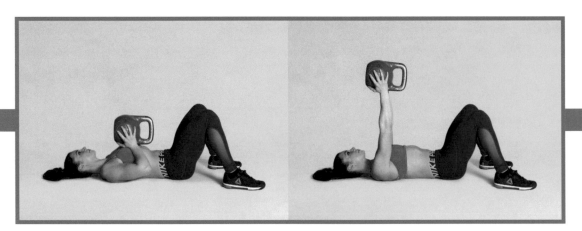

Chest Press Variation

Set up for the push-up by placing the hands shoulder width apart or slightly wider. Make sure the fingers are pointed forward. Squeeze the shoulder blades together and start the decent to the floor. The elbows should track straight back or at a 45-degree angle. Squeezing your glutes will keep tension in the core and aid in keeping the proper position. As you press out of the bottom of the push-up, do not change your body position.

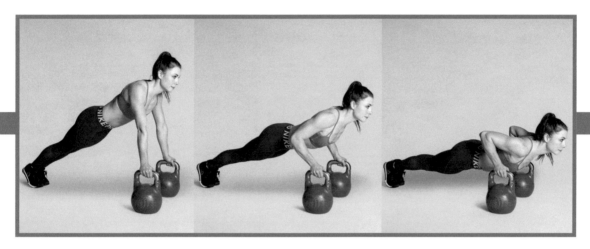

Push-Up

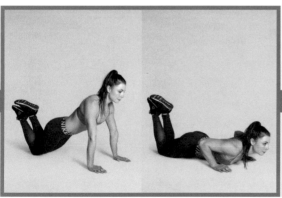

Knee Push-Up

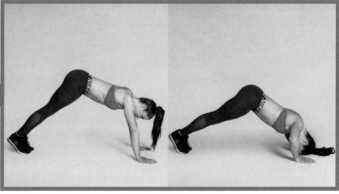

Pike Push-Up

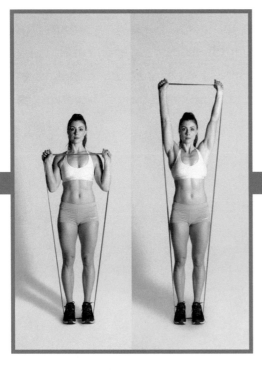

Banded Press

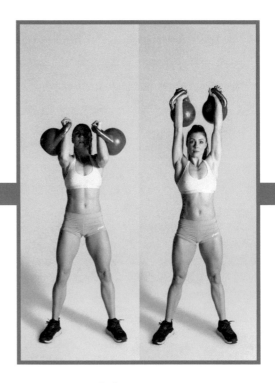

Double KB Press

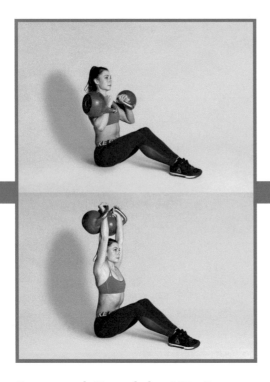

Seated Double KB Press

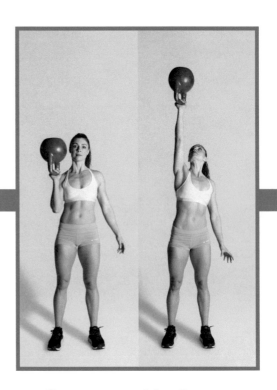

Bottoms-Up Press

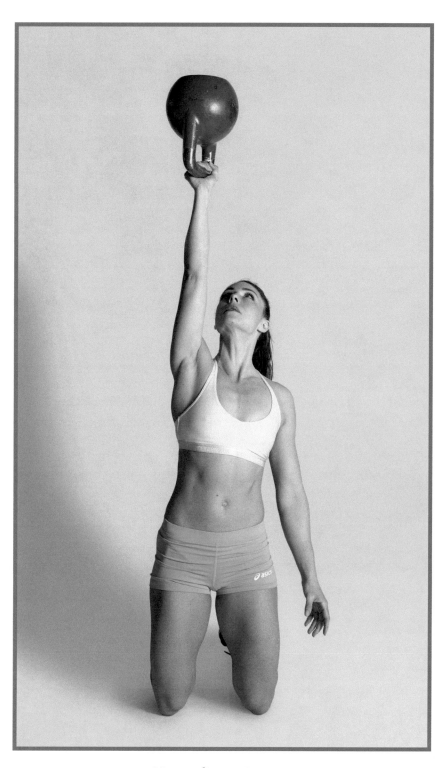

Kneeling Press

SWINGS

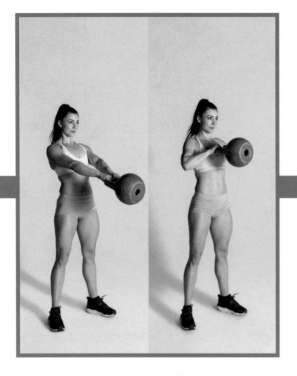

Swing Pull

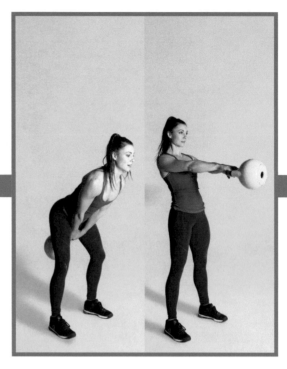

Two-Arm Swing

An "American style" swing is when the KB is brought all the way overhead

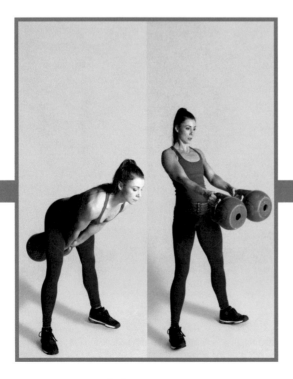

Double Swing

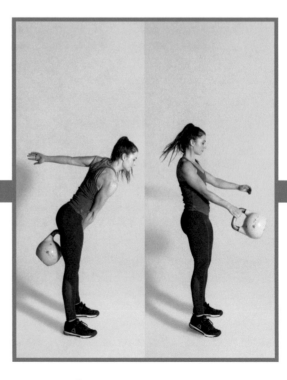

Single-Arm Sport Swing

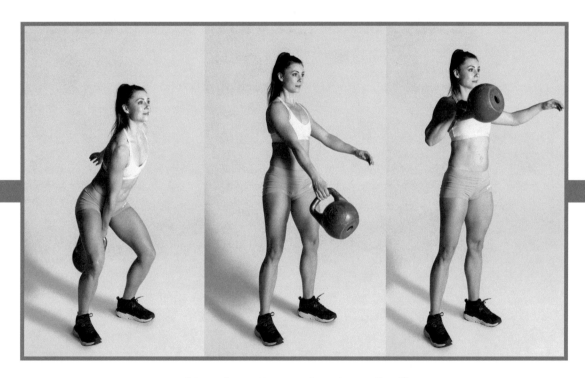

Single-Arm Swing Pull

ABDOMINAL

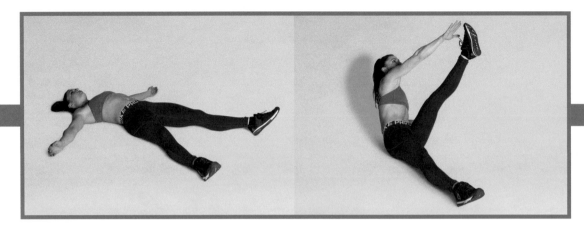

Starfish Crunch

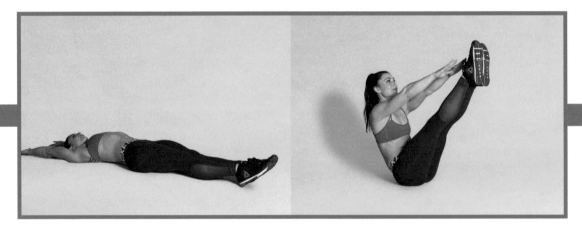

V-Up

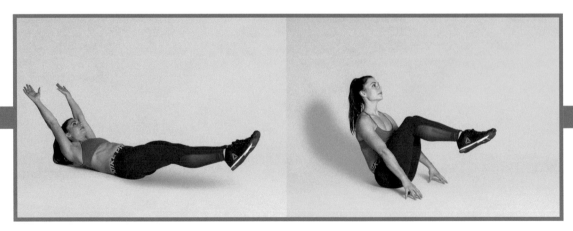

Tuck-Up

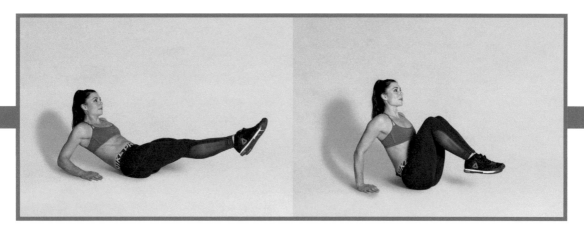

In and Out

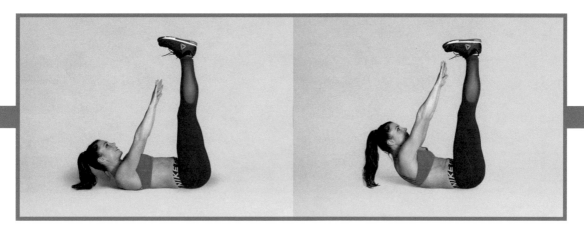

Toe-Touch Crunch

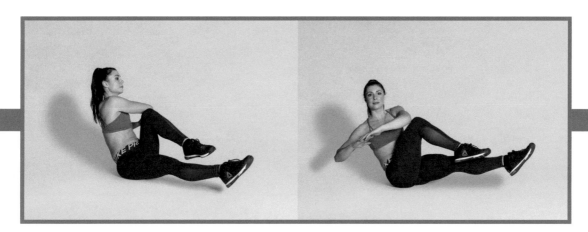

Bicycle Crunch

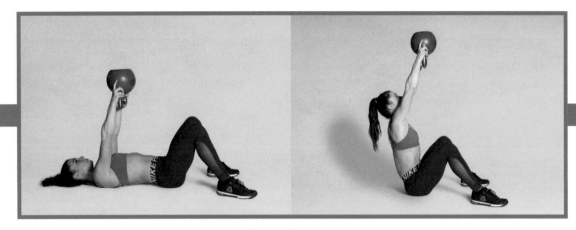

Weighted Sit-Up

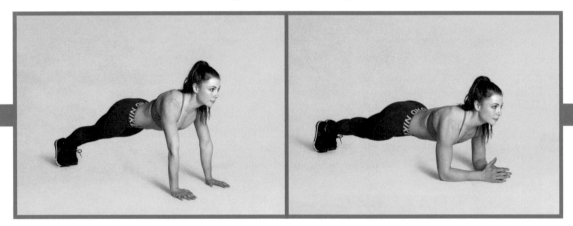

Plank Hold Variations

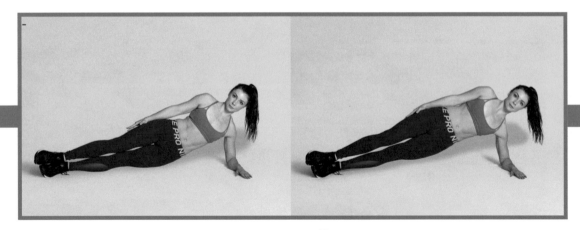

Hip Dip on Elbow

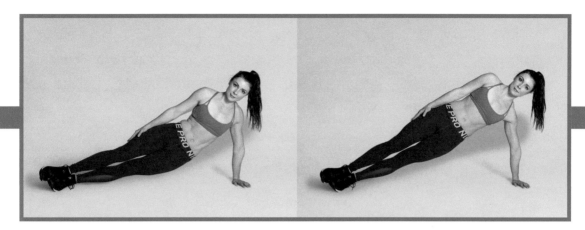

Hip Dip

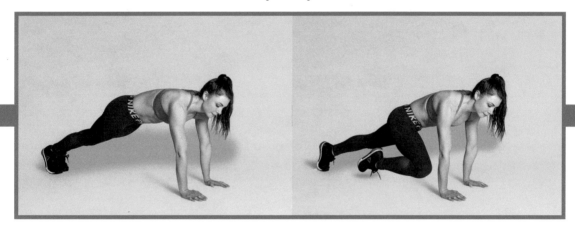

Mountain Climber

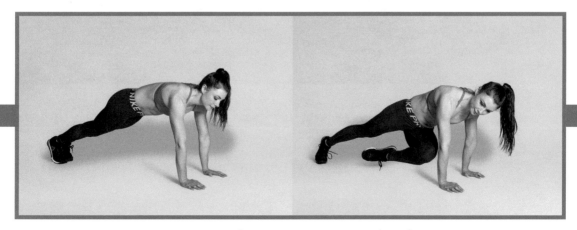

Cross Body Mountain Climber

NOTE: Keep the low back pressed against the floor and the chin tucked when doing ab exercises on your back. This keeps the abs more engaged and protects the low back. Paying attention to proper form and alignment is crucial in preventing injuries and maximizing the effectiveness of your abdominal workouts. Don't forget to breathe.

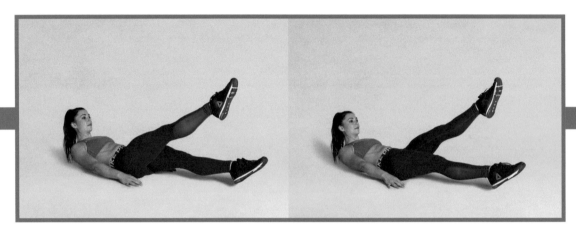

Flutter Kick

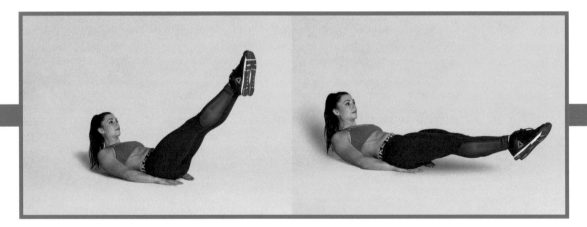

Leg Lowers

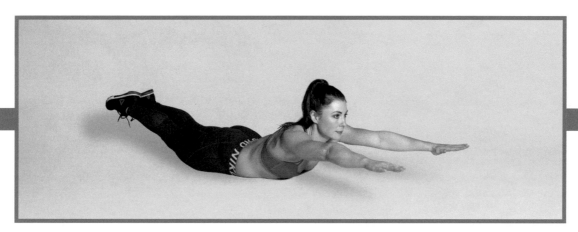

Arch Hold

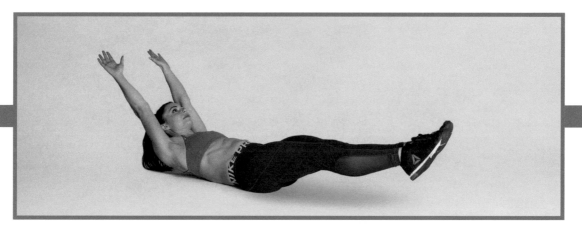

Hollow Hold

EXERCISES

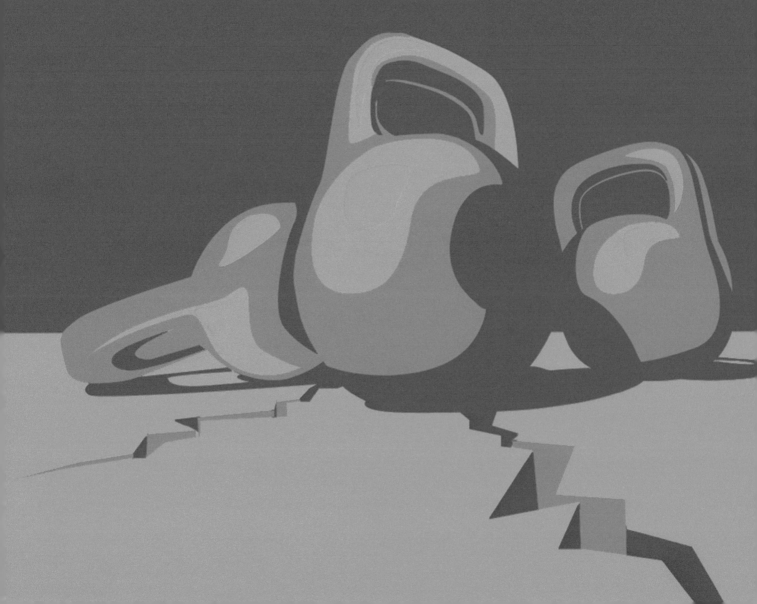

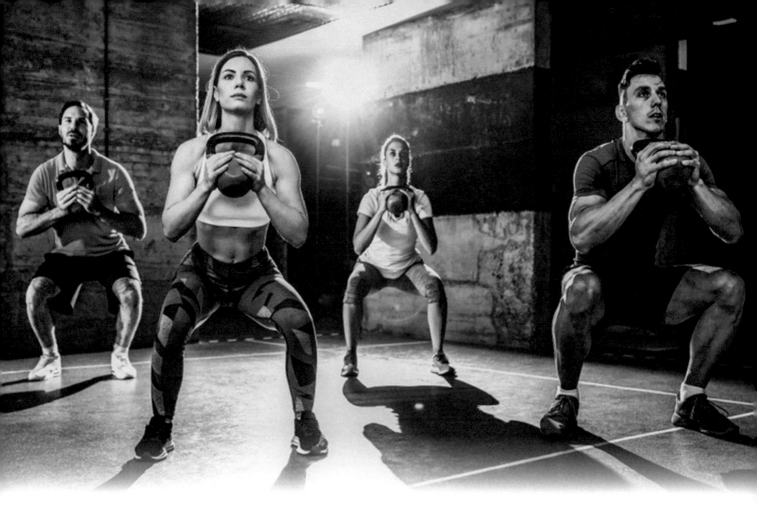

HOW TO USE ────── THE PROGRAM

Each day is broken into two sections: "KETTLEBELLS" and "ACCESSORY." The KETTLEBELLS section is related specifically to kettlebell sport exercises.

The ACCESSORY section is formulated to increase strength and build muscle. Some sessions have a cardio and/or a core workout to do after.

All the workouts are designed to be completed with one or two kettlebells and a resistance band. A variety of kettlebell weights is recommended to see maximum results.

This program can be used in multiple ways. On the next page are examples of how you could structure your week.

KETTLEBELL SPORT & FITNESS BASICS

Option 1

Day 1	Day 2	Day 3	Day 4
KETTLEBELLS - SESSION 1	ACTIVE REST / CARDIO	KETTLEBELLS - SESSION 2	ACTIVE REST / CARDIO
ACCESSORY - SESSION 1		ACCESSORY - SESSION 2	

Day 5	Day 6	Day 7
KETTLEBELLS - SESSION 3	ACTIVE REST / CARDIO	REST
ACCESSORY - SESSION 3		

Option 2

Day 1	Day 2	Day 3	Day 4
KETTLEBELLS - SESSION 1	ACCESSORY - SESSION 1	ACTIVE REST / CARDIO	KETTLEBELLS - SESSION 2
CIRCUIT OR BONUS WORKOUT			CIRCUIT OR BONUS WORKOUT

Day 5	Day 6	Day 7
ACCESSORY - SESSION 2	KETTLEBELLS - SESSION 3	REST
	ACCESSORY - SESSION 3	

Option 3

Day 1	Day 2	Day 3	Day 4
KETTLEBELLS - SESSION 1	KETTLEBELLS - SESSION 2	ACTIVE REST / CARDIO	ACTIVE REST / CARDIO
ACCESSORY - SESSION 1	ACCESSORY - SESSION 2		

Day 5	Day 6	Day 7
KETTLEBELLS - SESSION 3	CARDIO	REST
ACCESSORY - SESSION 3	CIRCUIT OR BONUS WORKOUT	

Active Rest: walking, leisurely bike ride, playing with kids or dog, yard work, cleaning, etc.

Cardio: running, biking, hiking, rowing, etc.

TERMS & WEIGHTS

AFAP = as fast as possible

AHAP = as heavy as possible

AMRAP = as many reps/rounds as possible

COMPOUND SET = two exercises of the same muscle group performed back-to-back with little or no rest between them

DL = deadlift

KB = kettlebell

OH = overhead

RDL = Romanian deadlift

RPM = reps per minute

SDHP = sumo deadlift high pull

SUPERSET = two exercises of opposing muscle groups performed back-to-back with little or no rest between them

Use the table below help you decide what weight kettlebell to use in the KETTLEBELLS section. This is only a guide, so use your discretion when picking your weight for each session. Adjust the weight based on your individual fitness level, gradually increasing it as you become more comfortable and proficient with the exercises. Listen to your body and prioritize form over lifting heavier weights to ensure a safe and effective workout.

Women	Novice	Intermediate	Experienced
Light	8kg	12kg	16kg
Medium	12kg	16kg	20kg
Heavy	16kg	20kg	24kg

Men	Novice	Intermediate	Experienced
Light	12kg	16kg	20kg
Medium	16kg	20kg	24kg
Heavy	20kg	24kg	32kg

HOW TO READ
THE PROGRAM

KETTLEBELLS				
Exercise	Weight	RPM	Time	Notes
Long Cycle	light	12-14	2/2 mins	rest 2-4 mins
Jerk (2 KB's)	medium	12-14	2 mins	

ACCESSORY				
Exercise	Weight	Sets	Reps	Notes
Squats (with KB - any style)	AHAP	5	8	
Reverse Lunge (with weight)	AHAP	3	16 (8/side)	
Skaters	AFAP	1	100 (50/side)	
OH Press	AHAP	3	8	use 2 KBs or do 8 each side
Chest Press	AHAP	3	10	use 2 KBs or do 10 each side
Hip Thrusts		3	30	
Arch Up Holds		3	20	

Exercise: the movement and how many kettlebells to use.

Weight: use the weight chart on the previous page to select the appropriate weight for your experience level.

RPM: the recommend number of reps per minute.

Time: the work time is written per hand or total. For example, 2/2 mins = two minutes per hand and 2 mins = two minutes total.

Sets: the number of sets to perform.

Reps: the number of reps to perform each set.

Notes: Rest times and any additional comments are here. Rest the indicated time between sets.

Example Flow:

Warm up.

Start your kettlebell training session with two minutes of single arm long cycle on each hand. Rest two to four minutes then do two minutes of jerks with two kettlebells. If you only have one kettlebell you will do two minutes per hand. After you complete the KETTLEBELL section, move on to the ACCESSORY section. Grab a kettlebell for squats. The kettlebell should be as heavy as you can tolerate for five sets of eight reps. Rest as needed between each set. Then, move on to the rest of the accessory work listed. Once you complete the accessory work, spend at least five to ten minutes stretching. Don't forget to log your workout!

WARM UP

Always warm up before beginning any workout to get your body prepared for physical activity. Warming up will help you perform the workout more efficiently and prevent injury.

5-15 mins: Start general - run, bike, jump rope, light KB swings, etc. (get your heart rate elevated)

3-5 mins: Spend a few minutes with light dynamic stretches (squats, boot strappers, good mornings, side lunges, etc.)

3-5 mins: Warm up the shoulders. See below for some shoulder warm-up exercises

3-5 mins: Lastly, start warming up for the kettlebell sets by doing the movement you're training with light weight and working your way heavier (to your working weight)

Some Example Shoulder Warm-Up Exercises:

- Band Pull-Apart
- Banded External and Internal Rotations
- Banded Rows
- Banded/PVC Pass Through
- Knee Push-Ups
- Light KB Swings and Swing Pulls
- Light OH Presses
- Scapular Push-Ups
- Windmills

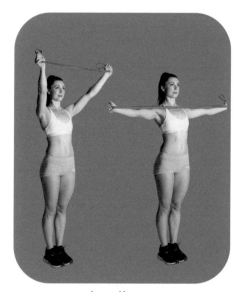

Band Pull-Apart

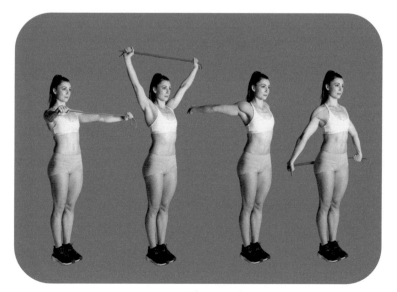

Pass Through

SESSION 1

KETTLEBELLS				
Exercise	Weight	RPM	Time	Notes
Long Cycle	light	12-14	2/2 mins	rest 2-4 mins
Long Cycle	medium	10-12	2/2 mins	rest 2-4 mins
Swing Snatch	medium	10-12	2/2 mins	one swing + one snatch

ACCESSORY				
Exercise	Weight	Sets	Reps	Notes
Squats (with KB - any style)	AHAP	5	8	
Reverse Lunge (with weight)	AHAP	3	16 (8/side)	
Skaters	AFAP	1	100 (50/side)	
OH Press	AHAP	3	8	use 2 KBs or do 8 each side
Chest Press	AHAP	3	10	use 2 KBs or do 10 each side
Hip Thrusts	-	3	30	
Arch Up Holds	-	3	20	

CARDIO	
Exercise	
5 ROUNDS:	
2:00 Run or bike	
10 Jump Squats	Note: increase jump squats by 5 reps each round

Notes: All kettlebell work in the KETTLEBELLS session is completed with one bell

2/2 mins = 2 minutes right arm + 2 minutes left arm.

Perform 2 minutes of the exercise for each hand, then, rest 2 to 4 minutes before performing the next set.

SESSION 2

KETTLEBELLS				
Exercise	Weight	RPM	Time	Notes
Jerk (2 KBs)	light	13-15	2 mins	rest 2-4 mins
Jerk (2 KBs)	medium	12-14	2 mins	rest 2-4 mins
Jerk (2 KBs)	medium	10-12	2 mins	rest as needed before moving on

ACCESSORY				
Exercise	Weight	Sets	Reps	Notes
Deadlift (2 KBs)	AHAP	5	8	
Sumo Deadlift (1 KB)	AHAP	3	12	
Bent Row (2 KBs)	AHAP	3	12	
Single-Arm Bent Row	AHAP	3	16 (8/side)	
Banded Bicep Curl	AHAP	3	15-20	
KB High Pulls (from hang)	light	3	15-20	use legs if needed
Swing Pull	light	1	100	as few sets as possible

CORE				
Exercise		Sets	Reps	Notes
Plank Hold		3	1-2 mins	
Crunches		3	30	

Notes: If working with only 1 kettlebell, do 2 minutes per hand.

If you don't have a band, pick another arm exercise or do one more set of bicep curls with KB.

See the "HOLDS" page for an example of the neutral grip.

113

SESSION 3

KETTLEBELLS				
Exercise	Weight	RPM	Time	Notes
Snatch	light	18-20	2/2 2/2 min	rest 2-4 mins after
Swings	heavy	any	1.5/1.5 min	
OH Walk	medium	-	1/1 min	hold KB in lockout position and walk

ACCESSORY				
Exercise	Weight	Sets	Reps	Notes
Reverse Lunge	AHAP	3	30 (15/side)	
Single-Leg Deadlift	AHAP	3	20 (10/side)	
Bulgarian Split Squat +Jump	AHAP	4	12 (6/side)	add a hop to the top of the movement
Push-Up	-	3	1 min	
Dips (chair, bench, KB)	-	3	15-20	keep elbows in tight
Single-Leg Hip Thrust	AHAP	3	40 (20/side)	

CARDIO	
Exercise	
3 ROUNDS:	
1:00 Squats	
1:00 KB Swings (light)	
1:00 Burpees	
1:00 Sumo Deadlift High Pulls	

Notes: All kettlebell work in the KETTLEBELLS session is completed with one bell. Use a chair, wall or bench for Bulgarian split squats; substitute split squats or lunges if needed.

SESSION 4

KETTLEBELLS				
Exercise	Weight	RPM	Time	Notes
Jerk	medium	12-14	1/1 min	rest 2 mins
Jerk	light	15-17	2/2 min	rest 3-4 mins
Long Cycle x 2 sets	medium	10-12	1/1 min	rest 2 mins between, as needed after
Swing + Clean	med/hvy	8-9	1.5/1.5	

ACCESSORY				
Exercise	Weight	Sets	Reps	Notes
Squats (with KB - any style)	AHAP	5	10	
Lunge (walking)	AHAP	4	16 (8/side)	
Side Lunge	AHAP	3	20 (10/side)	
OH Press	AHAP	3	10	use 2 KBs or do 10 each side
Chest Press	AHAP	3	12	use 2 KBs or do 12 each side
Hip Thrusts	AHAP	3	30	

CORE				
Exercise		Sets	Reps	Notes
Arch Up Holds		3	20	
Bicycle Crunch		2	40	
Plank Hold		2	max time	

Notes: All kettlebell work in the KETTLEBELLS session is completed with one bell.

SESSION 5

KETTLEBELLS				
Exercise	Weight	RPM	Time	Notes
Snatch	medium	17-19	2/2 min	rest 3-4 mins
Snatch	light	18-20	3/3 min	

ACCESSORY				
Exercise	Weight	Sets	Reps	Notes
Deadlift (2 KBs)	AHAP	5	10	
Sumo Deadlift	AHAP	5	12	
Bent Row (2 KBs)	AHAP	3	12	
Single-Arm Bent Row	AHAP	3	18 (9/side)	
Bicep Curl w/KB	AHAP	4	8-12	neutral grip
Banded Bicep Curl	AHAP	3	15-20	
Banded Reverse Fly	light	3	15-20	

CARDIO/CORE	
Exercise	
4 ROUNDS:	
1:00 Bicycle Crunches	
1:00 Sumo Deadlift High Pull [SDHP]	
1:00 Skaters	

Notes: All kettlebell work in the KETTLEBELLS session is completed with one bell.
If you only have one bell for the ACCESSORY work, go heavier and do the programmed reps on each side.

SESSION 6

KETTLEBELLS				
Exercise	Weight	RPM	Time	Notes
Swing Swing Snatch	medium	10	2/2 min	rest 1-2 mins
Swing Snatch	medium	12	1.5/1.5 min	rest 1-2 mins
Snatch	light	18-20	1/1 min	

ACCESSORY				
Exercise	Weight	Sets	Reps	Notes
Reverse Lunge	AHAP	3	30 (15/side)	
Standing Leg Extensions	-	3	30 (15/side)	flex quad 1 sec at top of each rep
Bulgarian Split Squat	AHAP	4	12 (6/side)	
Push-Up	-	3	1 min	2 sets regular, 1 set elbows in tight
Dips (chair, bench, KB)	-	3	15-20	
Single-Leg Hip Thrust	AHAP	3	40 (20/side)	

CARDIO/CORE	
Exercise	
3 ROUNDS:	
1:00 Jump Squats	
1:00 KB Swings (light)	
1:00 Squat Thrust/Up Down	

Notes: All kettlebell work in the KETTLEBELLS session is completed with one bell.

Add ankle weights to standing leg extensions if you wish. These can also be done in a wall-sit position.

The 'Squat Thrust/Up Down' is a no push-up burpee.

SESSION 7

KETTLEBELLS				
Exercise	Weight	RPM	Time	Notes
Jerk	light	14-16	2.5 min/2.5 min	rest 3-4 mins
Snatch	light	18-20	2.5 min/2.5 min	rest 3-4 mins
Long Cycle	med/hvy	9-10	2 min/2 min	

ACCESSORY				
Exercise	Weight	Sets	Reps	Notes
OH Press	AHAP	4	10	
Skull Crusher	med	4	12-15	
Band Pull Apart	AHAP	3	15-20	
Bottoms Up Press	AHAP	3	10 (5/side)	
Chest Press w/ Hip Bridge	med	3	12	lift hips while pressing
Hip Thrusts	-	3	30	
Thruster	med	3	20 (10/side)	

CORE				
Exercise		Sets	Reps	Notes
Starfish Crunch		2	30	
Arch Up		3	15	

Notes: All kettlebell work in the KETTLEBELLS session is completed with one bell.

SESSION 8

KETTLEBELLS				
Exercise	Weight	RPM	Time	Notes
Snatch	medium	17-19	2/2 min	rest 3-4 mins
Snatch	light	18-20	3/3 min	rest 1-2 mins

ACCESSORY				
Exercise	Weight	Sets	Reps	Notes
Deadlift (2 KBs)	AHAP	5	10	
Sumo Deadlift (1 KB)	AHAP	5	12	flex quad 1 sec at top of each rep
Bent Row (2 KBs)	AHAP	3	12	
Single-Arm Bent Row	AHAP	3	18 (9/side)	2 sets regular, 1 set elbows in tight
Bicep Curl w/ KB	AHAP	4	8-12	
Banded Bicep Curl	AHAP	3	15-20	
Banded Reverse Fly	light	3	15-20	

CARDIO/CORE	
Exercise	
4 ROUNDS:	
1:00 Bicycle Crunches	
1:00 SDHP	
1:00 Skaters	

Notes: All kettlebell work in the KETTLEBELLS session is completed with one bell.
If you only have one bell for the ACCESSORY work, go heavier and do the programmed reps on each side.

SESSION 9

KETTLEBELLS				
Exercise	Weight	RPM	Time	Notes
Swing Swing Snatch	medium	10	2/2 min	rest 1-2 mins
Swing Snatch	medium	12	1.5/1.5 min	rest 1-2 mins
Snatch	light	18-20	1/1 min	

ACCESSORY				
Exercise	Weight	Sets	Reps	Notes
Squat (with KB - any style)	AHAP	4	15	
1/2 Squat (fast pace)	-	3	30	squat above parallel and quickly
Single-Leg Deadlift	AHAP	4	12 (6/side)	
Runners Lunge	-	3	:30	rest :30 between sets
Hip Thrusts	AHAP	3	35	

CARDIO/CORE	
Exercise	
5 ROUNDS:	
20 Body Weight Squats	
30 Mountain Climbers	
40 High Knees	

Notes: All kettlebell work in the KETTLEBELLS session is completed with one bell.

SESSION 10

KETTLEBELLS				
Exercise	Weight	RPM	Time	Notes
Jerk (2 KBs)	light	13-15	3 mins	rest 2-4 mins
Jerk (2 KBs)	medium	12-14	2 mins	rest 2-4 mins
Jerk (2 KBs)	med/hvy	10-12	1 min	rest as needed after

ACCESSORY				
Exercise	Weight	Sets	Reps	Notes
Banded Press	AHAP	4	15	
Push Up	-	3	:30	rest :30 between sets
Seated Press	AHAP	3	15-20	
Chest Press	AHAP	4	10	
Banded Tricep Extension	AHAP	3	15	
Dips (chair, bench, KB)	-	3	15-20	

CARDIO/CORE	
Exercise	
3 ROUNDS:	
30 Lateral Jumps	
20 In and Outs	
10 Toe Touch Jumps	Note: Touch toes while squatting, then jump.

Notes: If working with only one kettlebell, do the recommended minutes per hand.

SESSION 11

KETTLEBELLS				
Exercise	Weight	RPM	Time	Notes
Swing Snatch	medium	10-12	2/2 min	rest 2-3 mins
Snatch	med/hvy	16-19	3/3 min	rest as needed
Single-Arm Swing	heavy		1/1 min	

ACCESSORY				
Exercise	Weight	Sets	Reps	Notes
RDL	AHAP	4	12	
Staggered Stance DL	AHAP	3	12 (6/side)	
Single-Arm Bent Row	AHAP	3	12 (6/side)	
Narrow Grip Row (1 KB)	AHAP	3	12	rest :30 between sets
12 Bicep Curl w/ KB	COMPOUND-SET - 3 SETS			
12 Banded Bicep Curl				

CARDIO/CORE	
Exercise	
Pick 1 Core or Cardio BONUS workout	

Notes: All kettlebell work in the KETTLEBELLS session is completed with one bell.

If you do not have a band pick another arm movement. See the upper body section above.

SESSION 12

KETTLEBELLS				
Exercise	Weight	RPM	Time	Notes
Long Cycle	heavy	10-12	2/2 mins	rest 2 mins
Long Cycle	medium	10-12	2/2 mins	rest 2-4 mins
Long Cycle	light	12-14	2/2 mins	

ACCESSORY				
Exercise	Weight	Sets	Reps	Notes
Walking Lunge	AHAP	3	30-20-10	30 reps total, 20 total, 10 total
Single-Leg Squats	-	3	10 (5/side)	
Push-Up	-	3	1 min	2 sets regular, 1 set elbows in tight
Dips (chair or bench)	-	3	15-20	
Hip Thrusts	AHAP	3	40	

CARDIO/CORE	
Exercise	
4 ROUNDS:	
20 Jump Squats	
20 Burpees	
20 KB Swing Pulls	

Notes: All kettlebell work in the KETTLEBELLS session is completed with one bell. The single-leg squats can be done onto a chair as a scale.

Test Week #1

Now that you've been training consistently for a few weeks, we'll test what you can do in 5 minutes for the snatch, jerk, and long cycle exercises. It's very important to write down your results so you can track and measure your progress.

The next 12 sessions will build on this program to bring you to closer to doing a 10-minute set. The program will continue to focus on the snatch, jerk, and long cycle equally.

Day 1: 5:00 Snatch @ medium weight
Day 2: 5:00 Jerk @ medium weight
Day 3: 5:00 Long Cycle @ medium weight

Feel free to work out after your test sets, but make sure you're recovered before the next test set day. You may want to consider using this week as a deload week and focus on these test sets, cardio, light weight movements and mobility.

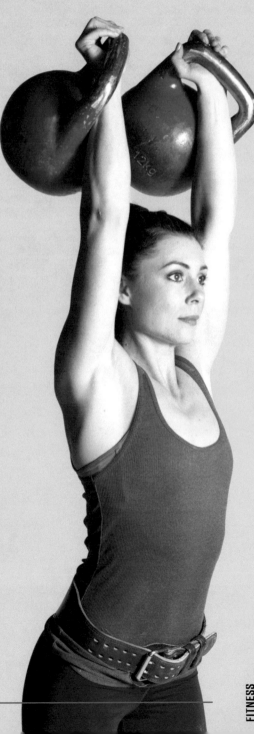

SESSION 13

KETTLEBELLS				
Exercise	**Weight**	**RPM**	**Time**	**Notes**
Snatch w/ :03 Hold Overhead	medium	n/a	3/3 min	rest as needed between
Swing Snatch	medium	12	2/2 min	

ACCESSORY				
Exercise	**Weight**	**Sets**	**Reps**	**Notes**
Squats (with KB - any style)	AHAP	4	15, 12, 10, 8	
Split Squat + Jump	AHAP	3	16 (8/side)	
Reverse Lunge + Knee to Chest	AFAP	1	100 (50/side)	
OH Press (1 KB Narrow Grip)	-	3	8	
Push-Ups on KB	-	3	12	
Single-Leg Hip Thrust	-	3	30 (15/side)	
Arch Up Holds - Elbow by Side	-	3	:30	

Notes: All kettlebell work in the KETTLEBELLS session is completed with one bell.

SESSION 14

KETTLEBELLS				
Exercise	Weight	RPM	Time	Notes
Long Cycle (2 KBs)	medium	8-9	2 min	rest 2 min
Long Cycle (2 KBs)	light	9-10	3 min	rest 3 min
Cleans (2 KBs)	medium	10-12	3 min	

ACCESSORY				
Exercise	Weight	Sets	Reps	Notes
Deadlift (any style)	AHAP	4	15, 12, 10, 8	
Sumo Deadlift (1 KB)	AHAP	4	15, 12, 10, 8	
Bent Row (1 KB)	AHAP	3	12	
Single-Arm Bent Row	AHAP	3	16 (8/side)	
Bicep Curl w/ KB	AHAP	4	8-12	neutral grip
Banded Bicep Curl	AHAP	3	20 ,15, 15	
Arch Up Holds - Elbow by Side	-	3	:30	

CARDIO/CORE	
Exercise	
10 minutes:	
10 SDHP	
20 Swing Pull	
20 In and Out	

Notes: All kettlebell work in the KETTLEBELLS session is completed with two bells.

SESSION 15

KETTLEBELLS				
Exercise	Weight	RPM	Time	Notes
Snatch x 5 sets	medium	18-20	2 min (1 min/hand)	rest 1 min between

ACCESSORY				
Exercise	Weight	Sets	Reps	Notes
Choose one of the workouts bellow:				
AMRAP 20				
5 Push-Ups	-			
10 Jump Squats	-			
20 Lunges	-			sub box jumps of step-ups if able
30 Sit-Ups	-			
or				
5 x 3-Minute AMRAPs of:				
3 Thrusters	AHAP			
6 Push-Ups	-			
9 Jump Squats	-			
rest 1 min between the 3 min sets				

Notes: All kettlebell work in the KETTLEBELLS session is completed with one bell.
If you only have one bell for the ACCESSORY work, go heavier and do the programmed reps on each side.

SESSION 16

KETTLEBELLS				
Exercise	**Weight**	**RPM**	**Time**	**Notes**
Jerk (2 KBs)	med/hvy	10	2 min	rest 2 min
Jerk (2 KBs)	med/hvy	10	2 min	rest as needed
Cleans	med/hvy	10	3 min	rest 2-3
Cleans	medium	10-12	3 min	

ACCESSORY				
Exercise	**Weight**	**Sets**	**Reps**	**Notes**
Squats	AHAP	4	12, 12, 10, 10	
Lunges (walking)	AHAP	3	30, 24, 20	reps are total
Curtsy Lunge	AHAP	3	20 (10/side)	
OH Press	AHAP	3	15, 12, 10	use 2 KBs or do reps per side
Chest Press	AHAP	3	15, 12, 10	use 2 KBs or do reps per side
Single-Leg Hip Thrust	-	3	30 (15/side)	

CORE				
Exercise		**Sets**	**Reps**	**Notes**
Arch Up Holds		3	:30	
Bicycle Crunch		2	40	
Plank Hold		2	max sets	

Notes: All kettlebell work in the KETTLEBELLS session is completed with two bells.

SESSION 17

KETTLEBELLS				
Exercise	Weight	RPM	Time	Notes
Swing Snatch	med/hvy	12	2/2 min	rest 3-4 mins
Snatch	light	18-20	3/3 min	

ACCESSORY				
Exercise	Weight	Sets	Reps	Notes
Deadlift (2KBs)	AHAP	4	15, 12, 10, 10	
Sumo Deadlift (1 KB)	AHAP	4	15, 12, 10, 10	
Bent Row (2 KBs)	AHAP	4	15, 12, 10, 10	use 2 KBs or do narrow grip rows
Single-Arm Bent Row	AHAP	3	15, 12, 10	per side
Bicep Curl w/ KB	AHAP	3	15, 12, 10	neutral grip
Banded Bicep Curl	AHAP	3	15-20	
Banded Reverse Fly	light	3	12-15	

CARDIO/CORE	
Exercise	
3 ROUNDS:	
30 Bicycle Crunches	
30 Sumo Deadlift High Pull	
30 Jump Squats	Note: Add weight if you can

Notes: All kettlebell work in the KETTLEBELLS session is completed with one bell.

If you only have one bell for the ACCESSORY work, go heavier and do the programmed reps on each side.

SESSION 18

KETTLEBELLS

Exercise	Weight	RPM	Time	Notes
Long Cycle (2 KBs)	medium	8-9	3 min	rest 3-4 mins
Cleans (1 KB)	heavy	10-12	3/3 min	

ACCESSORY

Exercise	Weight	Sets	Reps	Notes
Seated OH Press	AHAP	3	12-15	
Tricep Extensions	AHAP	3	12-15	
Banded Press	AHAP	3	15, 12, 10	Rest :30 between sets
Push-Up	-	3	1 min	
Dips	-	3	15-20	
Skull Crushers	AHAP	3	15, 12, 10	

CARDIO/CORE

Exercise	
3 ROUNDS:	
25 Jump Squats	
25 KB Swings	
25 Burpees	

Notes: If working with one bell, do 2 minutes per hand.

SESSION 19

KETTLEBELLS				
Exercise	**Weight**	**RPM**	**Time**	**Notes**
Snatch	med/hvy	16-18	2/2 min	rest 3-4 mins
Snatch	light	18-20	3/3 min	

ACCESSORY				
Exercise	**Weight**	**Sets**	**Reps**	**Notes**
Squats (with KB - any style)	AHAP	4	12, 12, 10, 8	
Split Squat	AHAP	4	12, 12, 10, 8	per side
Single-Leg DL	AHAP	3	20 (10/side)	
Single-Arm Bent Row	AHAP	4	8 (4/side)	
Wall Sit Leg Extension	-	4	12, 12, 10, 8	per side
Hip Thrust	AHAP	3	30	

CARDIO/CORE	
Exercise	
3 ROUNDS:	
20 Thrusters	
20 Starfish Crunch	
20 Arch Up	

Notes: All kettlebell work in the KETTLEBELLS session is completed with one bell.

SESSION 20

KETTLEBELLS				
Exercise	**Weight**	**RPM**	**Time**	**Notes**
Jerk x 10 sets	med/hvy	10-14	1 min	rest 1 min between sets

ACCESSORY				
Exercise	**Weight**	**Sets**	**Reps**	**Notes**
Deadlift (2 KBs)	AHAP	4	12, 12, 10, 8	
Sumo Deadlift (1 KBs)	AHAP	4	12, 12, 10, 8	
Banded Bent Row	AHAP	3	20	
Single-Arm Bent Row	AHAP	3	12, 12, 10, 8	per side
Banded Bicep Curl	AHAP	4	15-20	

CARDIO/CORE	
Exercise	
4 ROUNDS:	
1:00 Weighted Sit-Up	
1:00 Mountain Climbers	
1:00 Lateral Hops	

Notes: All kettlebell work in the KETTLEBELLS session is completed with two bells.

If working with only one bell complete the jerks as follows:

5 sets of 1 min + 1 min (rest 1 min between)

SESSION 21

KETTLEBELLS				
Exercise	**Weight**	**RPM**	**Time**	**Notes**
Snatch	med/hvy	16-18	8 mins	

ACCESSORY				
Exercise	**Weight**	**Sets**	**Reps**	**Notes**
Dips or Banded OH Extension	-	3	15-20	
Banded Reverse Fly	light	3	15-20	
Seated Press	AHAP	4	12, 12, 10, 8	
Renegade Row	AHAP	3	12-15	per side

CARDIO/CORE	
Exercise	
3 ROUNDS:	
:30 Arch Hold	
:30 Hollow Hold	

CARDIO	
Exercise	
5 ROUNDS:	
15 Push-Ups	
30 Mountain Climbers	
60 High Knees	

Notes: All kettlebell work in the KETTLEBELLS session is completed with one bell.

SESSION 22

KETTLEBELLS				
Exercise	**Weight**	**RPM**	**Time**	**Notes**
Jerk (2 KBs)	medium	10-14	1 min	rest 2 min
Jerk (2 KBs)	light/med	12-14	3 min	rest 3 min
Snatch	medium	16-18	3/3 min	

ACCESSORY				
Exercise	**Weight**	**Sets**	**Reps**	**Notes**
Squats (w/ KB - any style)	AHAP	4	12, 10, 10, 8	
Reverse Lunges (w/ weight)	AHAP	4	12, 10, 10, 8	per side
Runner's Lunge		3	12, 10, 10, 8	per side
Chest Press	AHAP	4	12, 10, 10, 8	
Hip Thrusts		4	30	

CARDIO/CORE	
Exercise	
3 ROUNDS:	
30 Flutter Kicks	
20 In and Outs	
10 Toe Touch Crunch	

Notes: Jerks should be completed with two bells, and snatch with one bell. If working with one bell on jerks, do the total time on each hand.

SESSION 23

KETTLEBELLS				
Exercise	Weight	RPM	Time	Notes
Snatch	medium	16-18	3.5/3.5 min	4-5 min rest
Long Cycle (2 KBs)	medium	8-9	2 min	rest 2-3 min
Long Cycle (2 KBs)	medium	8-9	2 min	rest 2-3 min
Swings	heavy	-	1/1 min	

ACCESSORY				
Exercise	Weight	Sets	Reps	Notes
RDL	AHAP	4	12, 10, 10, 8	
Sumo Deadlift	AHAP	4	12, 10, 10, 8	
Single-Arm Bent Row	AHAP	4	12, 10, 10, 8	per side
12 Bicep Curl w/ KB				
12 Banded Bicep Curl	CIRCUIT - 3 SETS			
12 Narrow Grip Row (1 KB)				

Notes: Snatch sets are performed with 1 bell. Long cycle should be done with 2 bells. If working with 1 bell, do 2 mins per side.

SESSION 24

KETTLEBELLS				
Exercise	**Weight**	**RPM**	**Time**	**Notes**
Jerk x 10 sets	light/med	12-15	2 min	rest 2 min between sets

ACCESSORY				
Exercise	**Weight**	**Sets**	**Reps**	**Notes**
Walking Lunge	AHAP	3	30-20-20	total
Wall Sit + Leg Extension	-	3	10 (5/side)	
Push-Ups	-	2	2 min	1 set regular, 1 set elbows in tight
Dips (chair or bench)	-	3	12	
20 Runner's lunge (10 each leg)	SUPER-SET - 3 SETS			
20 Hip Thrusts				

CARDIO/CORE	
Exercise	
4 ROUNDS:	
10 Burpees	
20 KB Swing Pulls	
10 Thrusters	

Notes: All kettlebell work in the KETTLEBELLS session is completed with two bells. If working with one bell, do 3 sets of 2 mins per hand.

Test Week #2

Now that you've been training consistently for a few more weeks, it's time to test what you can do in 7 minutes for the snatch, jerk, and long cycle exercises. Again, it's very important to write down your results so you can track and measure your progress.

You can repeat this program and change the weights, or you can find more programs at https://www.exercisestrength.com/products

If you choose to repeat this program use the same weights for the lifts you logged being an RPE 9-10 and compare how it feels the second time through. If a set was logged as an RPE 6-8 move up in weight.

Day 1: 7:00 Snatch @ medium weight
Day 2: 7:00 Jerk @ medium weight
Day 3: 7:00 Long Cycle @ medium weight

Feel free to work out after your test sets, but make sure you're recovered before the next test set day. You may want to consider using this week as a recovery week and focus on the test sets, light cardio, light weight movements and mobility.

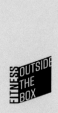

BONUS WORKOUTS

CORE/ABS

Core/Ab Circuit #1
5 Rounds x :30 each
Bicycle Crunches
Side Plank (R or L)
Side Plank (Other Side)
Mountain Climbers

Core/Ab Circuit #2
4 Rounds x :30 each (:10 rest)
In and Outs
Starfish Crunches
Plank Hold
Side Hip Dips (R or L)
Side Hip Dips (other side)

Core/Ab Circuit #3
3 Rounds x :45 each
Warrior Sit-Ups
V-Ups (sub In and Outs)
Flutter Kicks
Arch Hold
rest 1 min

Core/Ab Circuit #4
3 Rounds x 20 reps each
Slow Cross-Body Mnt Climbers
Flutter Kicks (20 each leg)

Core/Ab Circuit #5
3 Rounds x 15 reps each
V-Ups (sub: In and Outs)
Bicycle Crunches (15 each side)
Good Mornings (KB or Band)
Leg Lowers

Core/Ab Circuit #6
3 Rounds x 1:00 each
In and Outs
Hollow Hold
Arch Hold

Core/Ab Circuit #7
2 Rounds x 1:00 each
Plank Hold
Side Plank Hold (R)
Side Plank Hold (L)
Arch Hold
rest 1 min

Core/Ab Circuit #8
2 Rounds x 80 each
V-Ups (sub: In and Outs)
Bicycle Crunches

CIRCUIT TRAINING

Circuit #1
12 minutes - As many rounds as possible
5 Pull-Ups*

10 SDHP with KB

15 KB Squats

10 Burpees

5 Two-Hand Thrusters

* sub: Bent Rows with KB

Circuit #2
3 Rounds x 1 min each
KB Swings

Burpees

Side Shuffle (5-10 steps each side)

Circuit #3
5 Rounds (go heavy)
5 KB High Pulls

10 KB Swing Pulls

20 Mountain Climbers

Circuit #4
5 Rounds (heavy)
8 SDHP with KB

8 KB Deadlifts (narrow feet)

16 Step-Ups or Skaters

Circuit #5
20 Rounds for time
5 Deadlifts

5 SDHP

5 Burpees

5 KB Swings

Circuit #6
5 Rounds for time
10 Push-Ups

10 KB Swings

10 Jumping Lunges

Circuit #7
3 Rounds for time
30 Deadlifts

30 Jump Squats

30 Skaters

30 Push-Ups

Circuit #8
10 Minutes - As many rounds as possible
30 High Knees

30 Jumping Jacks

15 Burpees

15 KB Swing Pulls

CARDIO FOCUSED CIRCUITS

Circuit #1
For Time
1600m Run (1 mile)
300 Jump Ropes
800m Run (1/2 Mile)
150 Jump Ropes
400m Run (1/4 mile)

Circuit #5
5 Rounds Total
Run 2 mins at medium pace
Walk 1 mins
Run 2 mins at fast pace
Walk 2 mins
(35 mins total)

Circuit #2
2 Rounds for time
800m Run (1/2 Mile)
15 Burpees
100m Backwards Run
15 Burpees

Circuit #6
3 Rounds for time
800m Run (1/2 mile)
50 Lunges
50 Box Step Ups
rest 1 min

Circuit #3
15 Rounds
100m Sprint
rest 1 min

Circuit #7
20 Minutes
Run 2 mins at slow pace
Run :30 fast

Circuit #4
For Time
20 Squats
40 Mountain Climbers
Run 2 mins
20 Lunges (alternating)
40 Jumping Jacks
Run 2 mins
20 Burpees
40 V-Ups
Run 2 mins

Circuit #8
For Time
Run 200m (1/8 mile)
50 KB Swings
Run 400m (1/4 mile)
40 KB Swings
Run 200m
30 KB Swings
Run 400m
20 KB Swings

STRETCHING

We all need a minimum level of flexibility and mobility to go through our day. And most of us have at least just enough to meet life's daily demands. But over time, steady and limited range-of-motion activities can create shortened muscles. And shortened muscles can eventually lead to injury. For example, the hip flexors can become shortened after long periods of sitting or driving a car (Do much of that? Who doesn't?!).

Any activity that contracts the hip flexors over a reduced range of motion can cause the hip flexors to shorten. Even weight training exercises repeatedly performed in a shortened range of motion can lead to shortening of the psoas and Iliacus (hip flexors). Shortened muscles are one of the first steps leading to injury. Tight hip flexors can also lead to diminishment of the lordotic curve of the lumbar spine. A reduction of lordotic curve can impair the spine's load-bearing and shock-absorption capacity. When the spine cannot function normally, watch out! Tight hamstrings can have the same effect on the lumbar spine as hip flexors.

As another example, tight quadriceps can pull the patella (kneecap) upward, causing it to track abnormally. This can potentially result in a roughening of the underside of the patella, leading to pain and inflammation. The list of tight muscles facilitating imbalances can be endless! But don't worry, there are a few stretches you can do just about anywhere to help keep your muscles from getting too tight.

Static stretching (holding a stretch for a prolonged period) is commonly done post-workout, dynamic stretching (active movements that take your body through a full range of motion) can be beneficial before a workout to prepare the muscles for activity. Stretching should always be done with proper technique and within a pain-free range of motion to avoid injury.

Quick note: before stretching, it's a good idea to warm up. Your warm-up can be passive (hot bath or shower) or active (brief muscular activity). An active warm-up is preferred because it raises your core temperature and makes the target muscle tissues less viscous, which facilitates lengthening. Aim to sustain each stretch for a minimum of one minute, ensuring you focus on relaxation and controlled breathing throughout the stretching routine.

EXAMPLE STRETCHES

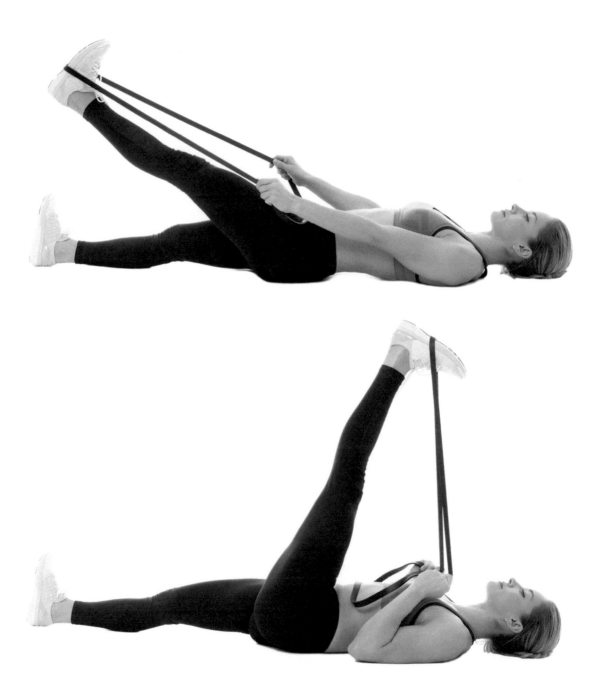

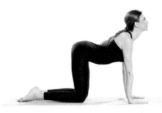
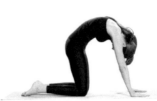
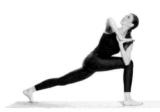

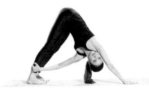

STRETCH
BEFORE AND
AFTER TRAINING
TO KEEP YOUR
BODY FEELING ITS
BEST

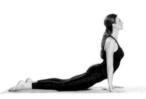

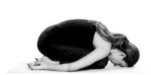
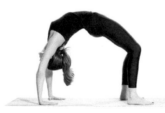
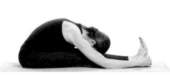

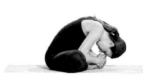
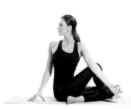
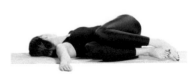

FAQs

Q: My grip keeps failing, and I'm having a hard time completing my KB sets. What should I focus on or do?

A: You'll get the most improvement by focusing on perfecting the cast, lockout, and back-swing. No amount of strength or conditioning can take the place of proper technique.

<u>Cast</u>: Make sure the bell isn't pulling on the shoulder (keep it seated and absorb the weight with the legs).

<u>Lockout</u>: Hands needs to be fully inserted, and the forearm/fingers need to be as relaxed as possible. Work on OH holds, OH walks, and OH lunges, and make sure your insertion and hand position is where it should be.

<u>Back-swing</u>: Be patient and let the bell come forward on its own before initiating the pull. Do lots of swings! Practice using the reverse hook grip, and make sure that the KB is tight to the body and the arm stays tight for as long as possible.

Q: Is it okay to use wrist protection?

A: Most competitions have specific requirements for wrist protection, but in training you can wear whatever you prefer. I recommend wearing something as you learn the proper positions to avoid discomfort and bruising. There are kettlebell-specific guards you can buy online with plastic inserts or you can use an elastic bandage. Elastic bandages can be found at your local pharmacy or grocery store.

Q: The KB keeps banging my arm when I'm doing the snatch and/or cleans. What am I doing wrong?

A: You may be gripping the bell too tight, inserting the hand at the wrong time, or flipping the bell too much before insertion. The grip should be completely loose so that the hand can be inserted with ease. As you can see on the next page, the insertion of the hand on the snatch starts well before the arm is overhead. If you start inserting the hand once your arm is close to reaching fixation (rack or overhead) it is too late.

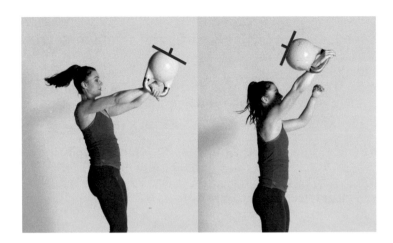

The bottom of the bell should be facing up as soon as you insert the hand. It should be facing back before your arm is by your ear.

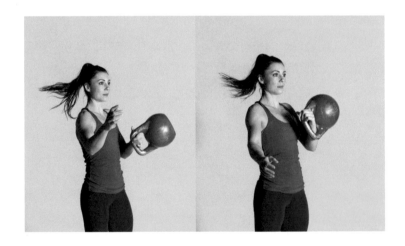

Notice how the hand is inserted before rack fixation occurs.

Q: What are the benefits of training with kettlebells?

A: Kettlebell training offers a low-impact way to work the entire body. Kettlebell exercises increase your mobility, explosive power, and athletic performance. Working with kettlebells also increases your mental tenacity due to the demand of coordination and body awareness needed for many of the movements.

Q: Can kettlebell training replace traditional weightlifting?

A: While kettlebell training offers a unique and effective approach to building strength and increasing conditioning, it may not completely replace traditional weightlifting. Kettlebells are excellent for dynamic movements, functional strength, and cardiovascular conditioning. However, traditional weightlifting can allow for more specific muscle isolation and heavier loads. Integrating both modalities into a well-rounded fitness routine will provide comprehensive benefits, targeting various muscle groups and enhancing overall physical fitness.

Q: Should I use chalk?

A: It isn't required but I do recommend it. Most lifters chalk not only their hands but the kettlebell too. Chalk helps you hang on to the kettlebell without having to squeeze it harder. The looser you grip the bell the longer it will take for your forearms to become fatigued.

Q: Should I use a lifting belt?

A: Wearing a belt is a personal preference. Most people will only wear a belt for Jerk and Long Cycle. A belt may be worn to provide stability to the back during training or, more commonly, use it to provide a place to rest or set the elbows on while in the rack position. A belt is usually worn low, across the hips, or at the waist. Lifters with better mobility or the ability to rest their elbows on the iliac crest of the pelvis may prefer to wear it in the low position. Lifters that aren't able to get their elbows on the iliac crest will wear the belt at their waist to create a base for the elbows. A solid base will allow for the efficient transfer of power from the legs. Figure out what works best for you.

KETTLEBELL SPORT & FITNESS BASICS

Q: What are the best shoes to wear?

A: Shoe selection is personal preference. At the very least, you want to wear a flat bottom shoe. Many lifters will wear weightlifting shoes while performing the sport movements. Weightlifting shoes have a hard sole which creates a stable base for maximum energy return. Having shoes with too much cushion, like a running shoe, absorb some of the energy that could be transferred to moving the weight.

Q: How can I use this program if I work out at a gym?

A: All of the accessory movements can be substituted using barbells, dumbbells and cable machines.

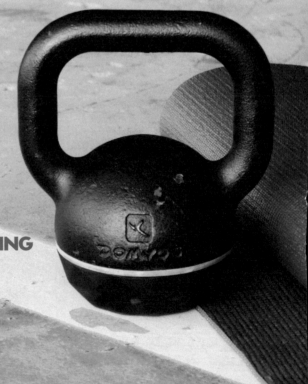

FOLLOW ME FOR UPDATES, KETTLEBELL SPORT CONTENT AND JUST TO STAY IN TOUCH. I LOOK FORWARD TO CONNECTING WITH YOU!

Instagram: @audreyburgio
www.youtube.com/itsjustcause
www.exercisestrength.com

WORKOUT LOG

Date	
Warm Up	

KETTLEBELLS

Exercise	Weight	RPM	Time	RPE/HR/Notes

ACCESSORY

Exercise	Weight	Sets	Reps	Notes

CARDIO/CORE

Exercise	

Additional Notes:	

NOTES

NOTES

KETTLEBELL SPORT & FITNESS BASICS